Tumor Angiogenesis and Modulators

Edited by Ke Xu

Published in London, United Kingdom

Tumor Angiogenesis and Modulators
http://dx.doi.org/10.5772/intechopen.95139
Edited by Ke Xu

Contributors
Daizo Yoshida, Akira Teramoto, Alok Chandra Bharti, Joni Yadav, Nikita Aggarwal, Arun Chhokar, Kulbhushan Thakur, Apoorva Chaudhary, Tanya Tripathi, Divya Janjua, Suhail Chhakara, Dikkshita Baruah, Anna Senrung, Gordana D. Radosavljević, Jelena Pantic, Bojana Simovic Markovic, Nebojša Arsenijević, Kanthesh M. Basalingappa, Pooja G. Singh, B.V Sushma, T.S. Gopenath, Rowyda Nawwaf Al-Harithy, José Manuel García-Castellano, David García-Padrón, Nerea Martínez-Aragón, Margarita Ramírez-Sánchez, Vicente Vera-Gutiérrez, Leandro Fernández-Pérez, Darmadi Darmadi, Riska Habriel Ruslie, Cennikon Pakpahan, Gvantsa Kharaishvili

First published in London, United Kingdom, 2022 by IntechOpen
IntechOpen is the global imprint of INTECHOPEN LIMITED, registered in England and Wales, registration number: 11086078, 5 Princes Gate Court, London, SW7 2QJ, United Kingdom

British Library Cataloguing-in-Publication Data
A catalogue record for this book is available from the British Library

Additional hard and PDF copies can be obtained from orders@intechopen.com

Tumor Angiogenesis and Modulators
Edited by Ke Xu
p. cm.
Print ISBN 978-1-80355-834-9
Online ISBN 978-1-80355-835-6
eBook (PDF) ISBN 978-1-80355-836-3

Meet the editor

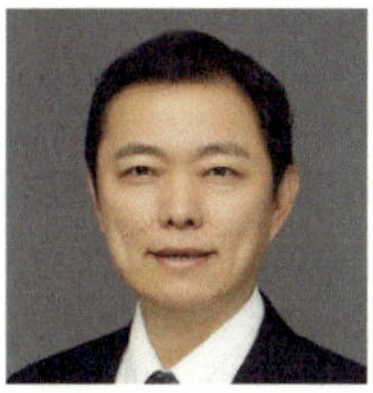

Professor Ke Xu earned his BSc in Microbiology from Nankai University, China, and his Ph.D. in Cell and Molecular Biology from the University of Essex, UK. He completed his postdoctoral training at the Institute of Cancer Research, UK, working on leukemia. Professor Xu carried out his research fellowship at Imperial College London, UK, investigating gene targeting and lung cancer. He joined the Tianjin Lung Cancer Institute of Tianjin Medical University General Hospital, China, in 2007 as a principal investigator to establish an independent research group studying the mechanism underlying cancer metastasis and chemoresistance. Professor Xu is an active member of the American Association for Cancer Research, the European Association for Cancer Research, and the American Society for Cell Biology.

Contents

Preface

Cancer is one of the leading causes of death worldwide. Tumor angiogenesis, the development and growth of blood vessels, plays a crucial role in tumor progression. The hypothesis of tumor angiogenesis was first proposed by Dr. Judah Folkman in 1971, and tumor angiogenesis has since become one of the most important fields in cancer research. When tumor mass reaches a size of 0.2–2.0 mm in diameter, it becomes hypoxic and loses nutrients, which limits its growth. This stimulates angiogenesis and the newly formed blood vessels deliver nutrients and remove metabolic waste from the tumor cells. Neovascularization involves several mechanisms, including sprouting angiogenesis, intussusceptive angiogenesis, vasculogenesis, recruitment of endothelial progenitor cells, vascular mimicry, and trans-differentiation of cancer stem cells. The tumor microenvironment promotes tumor angiogenesis via angiogenic factors, cytokines, non-coding RNA, and hypoxia. Tumor angiogenesis plays a vital role in tumor growth, especially in tumor invasion and metastasis. This book provides broad coverage of the field of tumor angiogenesis.

In Section 1, "Tumor Angiogenesis in Cancer", Chapter 1 reviews the research history of breast tumor neovascularization in both in situ and invasive breast cancer, the processes by which it occurs, and the impact of the microenvironment on neovascularization. It focuses on the factors that promote angiogenesis including hypoxia and vascular endothelial growth factor (VEGF) and the mechanisms of angiogenesis. Despite that pituitary tumors have been found to be less vascularized than normal pituitary tissue, accumulating evidence has shown that angiogenesis also plays an important role in pituitary tumors. In Chapter 2, the authors discuss several genes involved in angiogenesis. Hypoxia-inducible factors (HIFs) react to hypoxia and stress and maintain oxygen homeostasis, which influences development, metabolism, inflammation, and tumor progression. Endocan was induced by VEGF-A via phosphorylation and activation of VEGFR-2. Endocan promotes cell migration and tube formation during VEGF-A–mediated tumor angiogenesis.

In Section 2, "Modulators of Tumor Angiogenesis", Chapter 3 shows how tumor-derived exosomes play a significant role in tumor progression by accelerating angiogenesis. In this chapter, the authors introduce the exosome biogenesis, exosomal content, and mechanisms involved in exosome-induced angiogenesis in various types of cancers, including glioblastoma, breast cancer, lung cancer, and pancreatic cancer. They also discuss the therapeutic potential of tumor exosomes in angiogenesis. Chapter 4 reviews the sequence of morphological events that occur during neo-angiogenesis and the chemical mediators involved in this process, in particular the role of the IL-6/JAK/STAT signaling pathway in the control of these mediators. It also discusses estrogen intervention in this control procedure. This provides useful information for developing novel antitumor therapies. Chapter 5 reviews the functions of galectin-3 and IL-17 in tumor progression through their impacts on angiogenesis. Galectin-3 orchestrates practically all critical events during angiogenic cascade through interaction with various ligands and their downstream signaling pathways. Galectin-3 shapes the chronic inflammatory tumor microenvironment that is closely related to angiogenesis by sharing common signaling cascades and molecules. IL-17 contributes to tumorigenesis and progression via promoting critical events such as angiogenesis and the creation of an immunosuppressive milieu. Chapter 6 discusses the role of VEGF in liver disease. Liver diseases cause inflammation and hypoxia, which increase VEGF levels. The high VEGF level promotes the risk of chronic liver diseases and is associated with progressive disease course and poorer outcomes. Thus, VEGF is a promising modality for diagnosing liver cirrhosis and hepatic cell carcinoma (HCC). It may also be utilized to predict the outcome of liver cancer and to monitor the therapeutic response of patients. Chapter 7 examines the role of adipocytokines, which are a family of enzymes, hormones, growth factors, proteins, and other bioactive molecules that are important regulators of many processes. Adipocytokines are predominantly produced by pre-adipocytes and mature adipocytes to act through a network of autocrine, paracrine, and endocrine pathways. Leptin (LEP) is the first discovered adipocytokine. In angiogenesis, LEP acts directly as an endothelial growth factor or indirectly through cellular pathways such as STAT3/ERK1/2, JAK2/STAT3, MAPK/ERK, PI3K/AKT, p38, p53, MAPK, and Wnt/β-catenin. Chapter 8 investigates the role of the extracellular matrix (ECM) in tumor angiogenesis. ECM undergoes turnover and physiological remodeling, and during inflammation, experiences wound repair and tumor invasion. Remodeling of the ECM is an integral component of the angiogenic process and depends on the composition of matrix molecules, soluble pro-angiogenic and anti-angiogenic factors, and their spatial regulation. This chapter focuses on the myriad roles of those molecules and emphasizes their involvement in critical points of angiogenesis.

Despite significant progress in the study of tumor angiogenesis, the mechanism underlying tumor angiogenesis is still not fully elucidated. It is believed that based on new achievements in tumor angiogenesis research, as well as the rapid development of novel technologies, more cancer patients will benefit from new treatment strategies targeting tumor angiogenesis. This book is a useful resource in this regard.

Ke Xu
Tianjin Lung Cancer Institute,
Tianjin Medical University General Hospital,
Tianjin, China

Section 1

Tumor Angiogenesis in Cancer

Chapter 1

Tumour Angiogenesis in Breast Cancer

Pooja G. Singh, Kanthesh M. Basalingappa, T.S. Gopenath and B.V. Sushma

Abstract

Since the last comprehensive assessment of antiangiogenic therapy was published in Breast Cancer Research 3 years ago, clinical trials in a variety of tumour types, including breast cancer, have underscored the key relevance of tumour neovascularization. Bevacizumab, a drug designed to target vascular endothelial cell growth factor, was utilised in many of these studies (VEGF). Clinical trials using antiangiogenic treatment in breast cancer have highlighted the critical role of tumour neovascularization. Personalised medicine will become increasingly important to generate maximum therapeutic benefit to the patient but also to realise the optimal economic advantage from the finite resources available, according to a report by the US Department of Health and Human Services (HHS) and the National Institute for Occupational and Environmental Health (NIH). This overview covers the history of breast tumour neovascularization in both in situ and invasive breast cancer, the processes by which it occurs, and the impact of the microenvironment, with a focus on hypoxia. The regulation of angiogenesis, as well as the antivascular drugs employed in antiangiogenic dosing schedules, both innovative and traditional, are discussed.

Keywords: angiogenesis, VEGF, breast cancer

1. Introduction

Cancer has the potential to spread to nearby or distant organs, posing a life-threatening threat. For the metastatic spread of cancer tissue, the growth of the vascular network is crucial. Angiogenesis and lymphangiogenesis are the processes by which new blood and lymphatic vessels originate.

Cancer has the potential to spread to nearby or distant organs, posing a life-threatening threat. Tumour cells can enter blood or lymphatic vessels, circulate through the intravascular stream, and then spread to a new location (metastasis) [1]. The growth of the vascular network is crucial for cancer tissue metastatic dissemination. Angiogenesis and lymphangiogenesis are the processes that result in the formation of new blood and lymphatic vessels. Both are necessary for the formation of a new vascular network that will provide nutrients, oxygen, and immune cells while also removing waste. In tumour vascularization studies, angiogenic and lymphangiogenic factors are gaining popularity.

1.1 Angiogenesis in cancer

Endothelial cells, epithelial cells, mesothelial cells, and leucocytes, as well as cancer cells and host cells, all release chemicals that aid in angiogenesis. Plateletderived endothelial cell growth factor (I'D-ECGF), plateletderived growth factor (PDGF).

Angiogenesis is a series of events that are triggered by microvascular endothelial cells. Angiogenesis and lymphangiogenesis are essential for tumour growth and metastasis, and are triggered by chemical signals from tumour cells in the early stages of development. In a prior study, Muthukkaruppan and colleagues [2] looked at how cancer cells behaved when they were placed in different parts of the same organ. Blood circulation was present in the iris, but not in the anterior chamber [2]. Cancer cells without blood circulation grew to a diameter of 1–2 mm^3 and then stopped growing when placed in an area where angiogenesis was possible, but they grew to a diameter of more than 2 mm^3 when placed in an area where angiogenesis was possible.

If there is insufficient blood flow, tumours can become necrotic or even apoptotic [3, 4]. Angiogenesis thus aids cancer progression. The neovascularization stage of tumour angiogenesis is one of four steps in the process. Local injury to the basement membrane occurs first in tissues. Destruction and hypoxia take place almost immediately. Angiogenic chemicals cause endothelial cells to become activated and move. Endothelial cells multiply and settle in the third step of the process. Angiogenesis is still influenced by angiogenic stimuli, according to the fourth point.

Every 1000 days on average, vascular endothelial cells divide [5]. When tumour tissues need nutrition and oxygen, angiogenesis is induced. Activators and inhibitors of angiogenesis regulate the process. On the other hand, increasing angiogenic factor activity is insufficient to enhance neoplasm angiogenesis. Negative regulators or vascular growth inhibitors must also be inhibited [6].

1.2 Breast cancer: tumour angiogenesis

Clinical studies in a range of tumour types, including breast cancer, have proven the vital role of tumour neovascularization in the 3 years after the last comprehensive review of antiangiogenic therapy was published in Breast Cancer Research [7]. Bevacizumab (AvastinTM; Genentech, South San Francisco, CA, USA) was utilised in many of these trials since it was particularly intended to target vascular endothelial cell growth factor (VEGF). Bevacizumab is a recombinant VEGF antibody that binds to all known isoforms of VEGF-A and blocks receptor interaction, inhibiting angiogenesis and tumour growth. It was made from a mouse monoclonal antibody that had been humanised. One of the successes of antiangiogenic treatment, which was first suggested by Judah Folkman more than 35 years ago, is the critical contribution of this angiogenic factor in controlling many of the processes involved in angiogenesis, as well as its importance as a paradigm for the rational design of an anticancer agent.

Because all tumours (including liquid tumours like leukaemias) are angiogenesis-dependent, angiogenesis is highly restricted in adults, the endothelium of the vessels is accessible, and any treatment would be amplified through subsequent tumour infarction, the antiangiogenic approach has always appealed to researchers. Furthermore, because endothelial cells are non-neoplastic and should have a stable genome, cancer resistance should no longer be an issue [8].

To grow larger than a few centimetres in diameter, breast cancer, like other solid tumours, requires the formation of new blood vessels (neovascularization). The extra veins not only supply more nutrients to the tumour, but they also provide possible pathways for tumour dispersal and metastasis [9].

Tumour-induced angiogenesis first develops in pre-invasive high-grade ductal carcinoma in situ. In this case, a distinctive ring of microvessels emerges around the ducts, which are packed with proliferating epithelial cells. As the tumour grows, the amount of neovascularization increases [10]. Increased microvascular density or development, as well as variables that encourage new vessel growth, have been associated to poor breast cancer prognosis.

As a result, a significant amount of study has been focused on identifying the factors in the tumour microenvironment that promote and maintain angiogenesis in the hopes of limiting neovascularization and, as a result, tumour development and dissemination. Furthermore, unlike tumour cells, which are genetically unstable and can develop resistance to many therapeutic medications fast, normal vascular endothelium lacks mutations that would allow drug resistance [11, 12]. Both research lines are investigated in this paper.

Although the presence of axillary lymph nodes is the most important prognostic marker in operable breast cancer, it does not entirely explain for the wide range of disease outcomes. More precise prognostic indications would aid in the identification of patients at high risk of illness recurrence and mortality who would benefit from systemic adjuvant therapy [13]. Microvessel density (count or grade) in invasive breast cancer (a measure of tumour angiogenesis) is associated with metastasis and so may be a prognostic sign, according to recent research.

Breast tumour growth requires angiogenesis, or the rapid formation of new blood vessels, in order to acquire enough oxygen and nutrients [14]. Breast cancer cells, like all other biological tissues, rely on a vascular network of capillaries to provide food and oxygen on a regular basis. Endothelial cells (ECs), which line the interior surface of blood vessels, do not reproduce, hence capillaries do not proliferate. Hypoxia (low oxygen) triggers a variety of transcriptional responses that are mediated by transcription factors called hypoxia-inducible factors (HIFs) [15–18]. HIFs are transcription factors that regulate the expression of genes involved in physiological processes like metabolism, angiogenesis, and cell division. Local angiogenesis is one of the tumour microenvironment's long-term major responses to low O2 levels [19, 20].

It is the fusion of EC precursors that leads to the creation of capillary plexus, which thereafter evolves into blood vessels. Angiogenesis is required for a variety of normal processes, including embryonic development, growth, and wound healing [21].

As a result, the tumour activates an angiogenic switch and enters an irreversible active angiogenic state. Because of the tumour's newly acquired status, it can recruit new capillaries, restoring oxygen and nutrients to both angiogenic and non-angiogenic cells, resulting in rapid tumour growth [9, 22–24]. Despite the fact that surgical excision of tumours is the current standard of care for breast cancer, adjuvant therapy, such as anti-angiogenic therapy, has been used after surgery in advanced disease stages when surgery is no longer an option [25].

Angiogenic growth factors, such as vascular endothelial growth factor (VEGF) and fibroblast growth factors, are primarily involved in the initiation and progression of tumour angiogenesis (FGF). Angiogenic factor levels, as well as the number of vascular networks created as a result, have been shown to predict breast cancer survival in many studies. To put it another way, high levels imply that the tumour cells are aggressive and are linked to a poor prognosis. The rate and degree to which blood vessels permeate are controlled by these variables in connection with beginning angiogenesis [26–29]. Angiogenesis-targeting compounds have recently received a lot of attention in breast cancer research.

Bevacizumab, a humanised anti-VEGF monoclonal antibody, has been the most extensively investigated molecule [30–33]. After promising results in preclinical trials targeting VEGF, the FDA authorised bevacizumab in 2008 for the treatment of metastatic HER2-negative breast cancer [34, 35].

Following that, multiple anti-angiogenic medicines targeting VEGF or blocking its receptor's action were licenced, and they are now routinely utilised in the treatment of various malignancies [36–40]. The FDA, however, revoked its certification in 2011 due to conflicting results from earlier trials and allegations of increased toxicity as a result [41–44].

While the discovery of these anti-angiogenic drugs and small molecules was heralded as a potential victory in one aspect of the cancer fight, the agents' modest activities, such as their inability to arrest recurrent tumours in a latent state and the moderate improvement in overall patient survival, dampened the celebration.

1.3 The angiogenic cycle

Endothelial cells in normal, quiescent capillaries are in contact with a laminin-rich basement membrane and a layer of supportive pericytes that is 1- to 2-cell thick. Angiogenesis necessitates the weakening of connections between nearby pericytes as well as the degradation of the basement membrane [45]. The integrin adhesion receptors help endothelial cells re-enter the cell cycle and infiltrate the surrounding stromal matrix. Endothelial cells begin to resynthesize a basement membrane, which aids in cell cycle exit and promotes the creation of a capillary-like morphology [46]. Pericytes are then recruited to newly formed capillaries to help mature arteries stabilise [47]. Chronic exposure to angiogenic factors in the tumour microenvironment that promote basement membrane proteolysis or antagonise endothelial–pericyte interactions leads to the formation of a relatively unstable, highly permeable network of vessels that does not fully mature but can supply nutrients to meet the tumour's growing metabolic demands. Increased arterial permeability is thought to encourage tumour cell extravasation and, eventually, spread [48, 49].

2. Factors that promote angiogenesis

2.1 Hypoxia

Hypoxia has long been suspected as a significant angiogenic stimulator within the tumour microenvironment. Densely packed, quickly proliferating cells with limited nutritional inputs are the source of low tissue oxygen tension [50]. In recent years, researchers have made tremendous progress in understanding the biochemical and molecular reactions to hypoxia, as well as how the tissue senses low oxygen tension [51]. It was discovered that the hypoxia-inducible factor (HIF), a heterodimeric transcription factor made up of the hypoxic response factor (HIF-1) and the constitutively expressed aryl hydrocarbon receptor nuclear translocator (ARNT or HIF-1), is particularly significant [52, 53].

HIF-1 binds to the von Hippel-Lindau (VHL) protein in oxygenated circumstances, causing ubiquitination and fast destruction [54]. In hypoxic settings, on the other hand, this factor is stabilised: it is unable to associate with VHL protein because prolyl hydroxylase, an enzyme that typically alters HIF-1 to facilitate its interactions with VHL protein, is inactive. As a result, the oxygen sensor has been proposed as prolyl hydroxylase [55–59].

Animals lacking HIF-1 had markedly reduced angiogenic responses, indicating that it plays a vital role in experimental tumour growth and tumour-associated angiogenesis. Human ductal carcinomas overexpress HIF-1, whereas benign tumours with little angiogenesis do not. In the hypoxic tumour microenvironment, stabilised HIF-1 induces the expression of a variety of proangiogenic mediators, including vascular endothelial growth factor (VEGF) and one of its receptors, VEGF receptor 1 (VEGFR1) [60–62].

2.2 Vascular endothelial growth factor

VEGF is a powerful and selective endothelium mitogen that can produce a rapid and full angiogenic response, as its name suggests. VEGF (VEGF-A), the most investigated and implicated in tumour-induced angiogenesis, is a family of glycoproteins (VEGF-A, -B, -C, and -D) that are linked to VEGF (VEGF-A). The lymphatic endothelium responds to VEGF-C and -D in a big way [63].

VEGF is produced and released by a range of normal cell types, but its expression is dramatically increased in tumour cells, including a variety of breast malignancies, as well as reactive breast tumour stromal cells [64]. In contrast to other cytokines produced by tumour cells, VEGF functions almost exclusively on endothelial cells because expression of the major VEGF receptor, VEGFR2, is confined to such cells. Interfering with VEGF or VEGFR2 allows for the specific targeting of tumour endothelium [65]. VEGFR1, on the other hand, is expressed by endothelial cells, monocytes, and macrophages, and its role was unknown until recently.

When VEGF binds to its receptor, it activates an intracellular signalling cascade that causes gene expression modifications that promote endothelial cell migration and proliferation [66]. Furthermore, because VEGF not only functions as an endothelium mitogen but also increases capillary permeability, it's not surprising that the leakiness of tumour arteries is a fundamental distinguishing feature.

2.3 VEGF and breast tumour angiogenesis

An increase in VEGF synthesis by tumour cells and cells in the tumour stroma has been connected to angiogenesis induced by breast tumours, as previously mentioned. VEGFR2 expression was also shown to be greater in the endothelial cells of the adjacent breast tumour. Indeed, higher VEGF expression correlates with the first detectable breast-tumour driven angiogenesis in pre-invasive high grade ductal carcinoma in situ [67].

The elevated expression of VEGF in the breast tumour environment is thought to be due to a number of causes. Hypoxia and HIF-1 are clearly important factors. The fact that premenopausal women had higher levels of VEGF expression than postmenopausal women suggests that steroid hormones may also boost VEGF expression [68, 69]. Estradiol has long been known to be angiogenic, and evidence suggests that oestrogen effects may be mediated through VEGF induction. In certain breast cancer cell lines, estrogens increase VEGF expression whereas progestins lower it. Tamoxifen, an oestrogen receptor inhibitor, has recently been found to reduce VEGF transcription. However, whether oestrogen receptor expression is linked to VEGF expression and vascular density has to be determined.

VEGF production is also influenced by changes in the tumour environment. Matrix metalloproteinases, for example, are frequently secreted by numerous tumour cells, including human breast cancers [70]. Matrix metalloproteinase (MMP)-9, which is produced by tumour cells and expressed at high levels in human breast cancers, is one member of this family that has attracted a lot of attention. MMP-9 has been found to proteolyze the surrounding extracellular matrix, releasing trapped VEGF and thereby enhancing its bioavailability.

The expression of HER2 is another significant alteration in breast cancers. HER2 is a tyrosine kinase receptor that belongs to the epidermal growth factor receptor family and is expressed by the ERB2 gene [71, 72]. It signals in the lack of a known ligand. Furthermore, HER2 overexpression or heregulin stimulation causes an increase in VEGF mRNA, whereas treatment of breast tumours with an anti-HER2 neutralising antibody inhibits VEGF synthesis in a dose-dependent manner. Furthermore, HER2 was found to boost the rate of HIF-1 protein production in a new, rapamycin-dependent mechanism, rather than by blocking degradation as seen during hypoxia [73, 74].

VEGF production can also be boosted by changes in epithelial gene expression linked to tumorigenicity. The 644 integrin, which typically facilitates connections between breast epithelium and basement membrane, is upregulated and mislocalized in breast carcinoma cells, promoting tumour cell invasiveness. According to recent research, 644 signalling causes the inactivation of eIF-4E, a translational repressor, which enhances VEGF translation and, in turn, tumour cell survival [75–77]. The 644 signalling pathway, which enhances VEGF translation, converges on a rapamycin-sensitive route, similar to the HER2-mediated increases in HIF-1 and VEGF. Importantly, the tumour cells' increased VEGF production has been shown to act in an autocrine manner, promoting epithelial cell survival directly.

2.4 Mechanisms of angiogenesis

Tumour development and metastasis are dependent on angiogenesis. Necrosis occurs when a tumour's blood supply is cut off, preventing it from growing. After a while, any further metastatic spread into the systemic circulation is stopped. Scientists have been studying angiogenesis and the different variables that regulate it in order to better understand how it affects breast cancer and develop a strategy to limit tumour progression [25, 29]. Because of the dual nature of this process, it's critical to understand and distinguish between normal angiogenesis processes, such as wound healing, normal growth, and embryo nutrition, and tumour-related angiogenesis mechanisms.

Angiogenesis, which involves communicating between tumour cells and a variety of other cell types within the tumour microenvironment, is initiated by some compounds known as angiogenic activators because of their capacity to stimulate cell proliferation in vitro. The generation of pro-angiogenic growth factors by tumour cells, which impact the existing vasculature, has been shown to be necessary for the induction of this process [21]. To generate and stabilise newly created blood vessels, a delicate signal balance between pro- and anti-angiogenic factors is vigorously maintained in the microenvironment during these closely regulated processes [78]. As a result, numerous investigations have demonstrated that these angiogenic activators are critical in the growth of malignancies.

Certain tumour cells express both pro- and anti-angiogenic proteins, which encourage and inhibit angiogenesis, according to previous research. Tumours are thought to turn on the angiogenic switch by reversing the balance of angiogenesis inducers and inhibitors [29, 37]. This switch can be made by altering gene transcription, as seen in various cancers where VEGF and/or FGF levels are higher than in healthy tissue. The levels of endogenous inhibitors are lowered in some cancers, on the other hand. The intricate mechanism that drives these alterations in the regulators' balances, on the other hand, remains a fascinating subject of research (**Figure 1**).

The tumours ability to switch on angiogenesis is determined by the balance of this switch. Further research revealed that a decrease in anti-angiogenic protein production activates the tumour angiogenic switch, promoting tumour growth and metastasis [79–81]. Stimulating angiogenesis in a tumour and forming the endothelial tubes that result is a multistep process governed by hypoxia at each stage. This pathway is heavily reliant on ECs expressing HIF-1, a heterodimeric transcription factor. Under hypoxic conditions, the HIF-1 protein is stabilised and forms a heterodimer with HIF-1, and this pair promotes the transcription of multiple target genes to adapt to the hypoxic environment in human cancer cells.

HIF-1, in conjunction with other members of the HIF family, has been demonstrated in certain studies to govern practically every element of angiogenesis, making the HIF pathway a master regulator of angiogenesis [82]. In various malignancies, HIF-1 and HIF-2 expression has also been linked to a poor prognosis and metastatic illness. As a result, it's regarded as a promising therapeutic target for a variety of medical conditions (**Figure 2**).

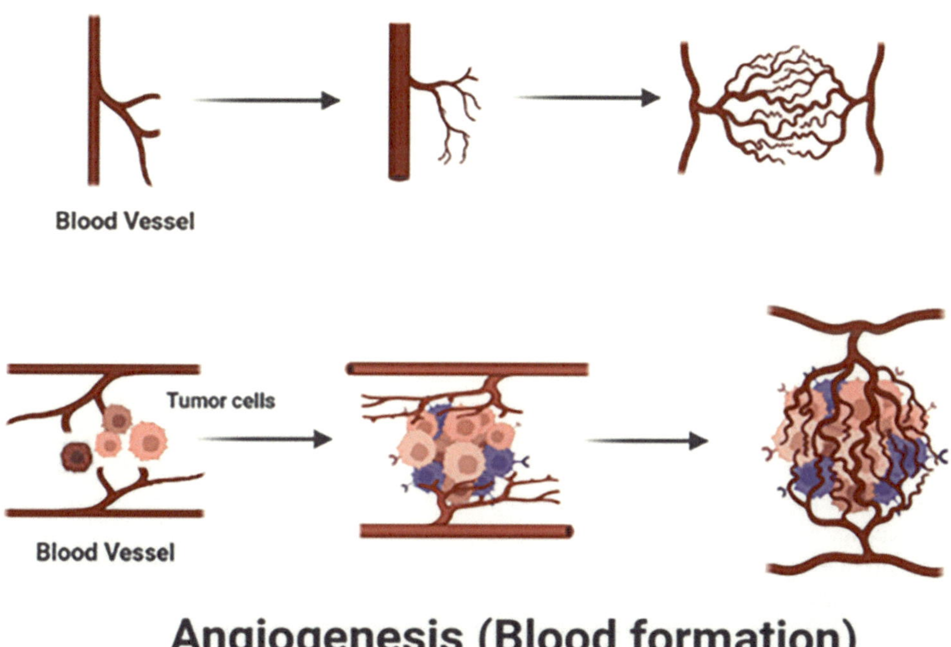

Figure 1.
Angiogenesis is a physiological process that results in the formation of new blood vessels from existing ones. From pre-existing capillaries, new blood vessels emerge. The tumour receives crucial nutrients for growth from the new blood vessels that have sprouted near and within the tumour. Angiogenesis in healthy tissues is regulated by a balance of anti- and pro-angiogenic factors (bottom), but the presence of angiogenic factors in tumours disrupts this balance, resulting in abnormal blood vessel structure and function, as well as hypoxia. The vasculature is normalised and the balance is restored.

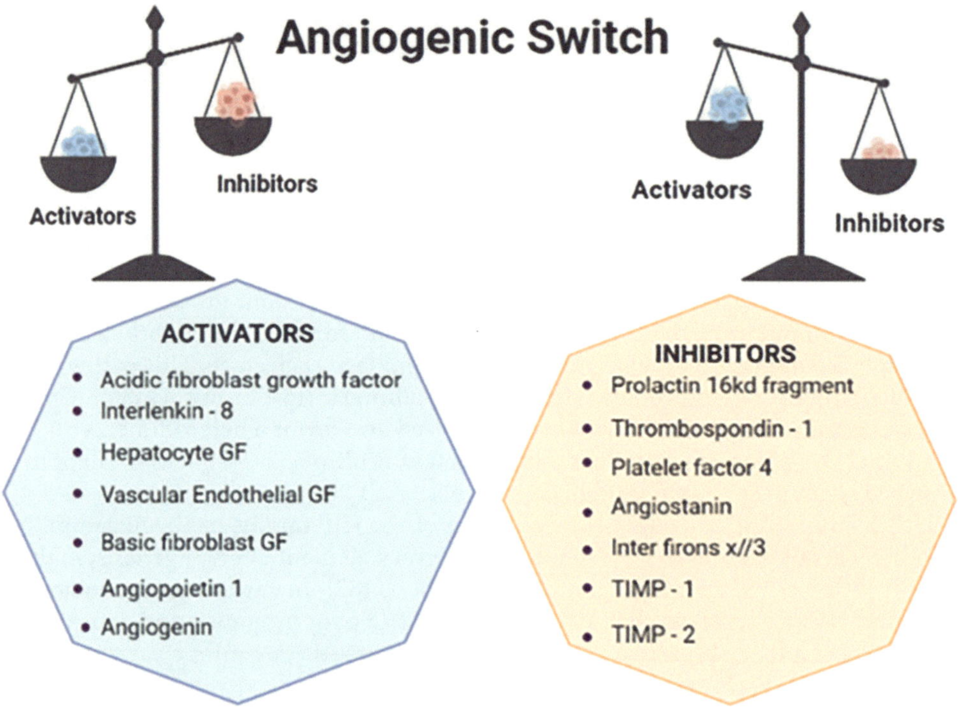

Figure 2.
This figure depicts the balance hypothesis of the angiogenic switch. Angiogenesis switch mechanism is assumed to be in charge of normal angiogenesis (formation of new capillaries). By utilising angiogenesis inducers and inhibitors, which flip the switch, this balance can be tilted in favour of enhanced blood vessel formation. Reduced inhibitor levels (thrombospondin-1, 16 kD prolactin, interferon, platelet factor-4, Angiostatin, and others) or increased activator levels (aFGF, bFGF, VEGF, and others) can tip the balance and activate the switch, resulting in the formation of new blood vessels.

Hypoxia and activation of the HIF pathway in cancer cells are required for the sprouting and formation of new blood vessels because they control the expression of several pro-angiogenic genes [83]. Some of the most powerful cytokines are VEGF, an endothelial mitogen and pro-angiogenic factor, angiopoietin-1, angiopoietin-2, platelet-derived growth factor (PDGF), and basic fibroblast growth factor (bFGF) [84–88].

The FGF and VEGF families of angiogenetic growth factors have gotten more attention than the others. In 1983, the protein VEGF-A (vascular endothelial growth factor) was identified and sequenced. It was the first cytokine to be identified as a key contributor to tumour angiogenesis, was purified from tumour cell ascites as vascular permeability factor (VPF), and was also revealed to have pharmacological effects on EC mitogenesis; consequently, VPF is referred to as VEGF (**Figure 3**) [89, 90].

In vivo and in vitro, VEGF is now known to be a multifunctional peptide capable of triggering receptor-mediated endothelial cell proliferation and angiogenesis. The VEGF family contains at least five members, each of which has three VEGF receptors (VEGFR) [91–93]. These receptors use transmembrane receptor tyrosine kinases to communicate with the cell's interior (RTKs). The VEGF gene is subject to complex transcriptional control, and four distinct RNA isoforms are produced with varying biological features as a result of alternative splicing of its pre-mRNAs. VEGF-B, VEGF-C, VEGF-D, VEGF-E, and platelet-derived growth factor are all produced as a result of this process (PDGF).

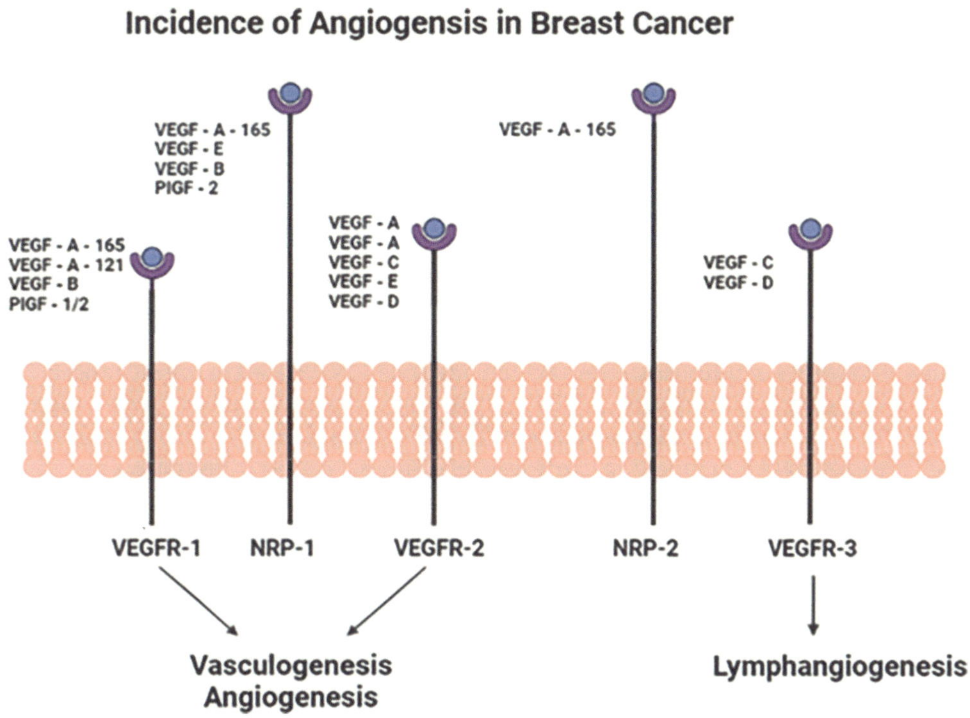

Figure 3.
This diagram depicts the receptor binding selectivity and signalling pathways of members of the vascular endothelial growth factor (VEGF) family. VEGF family members bind to VEGFR-1, VEGFR-2, and VEGFR-3 receptor tyrosine kinases, which activate a variety of signalling pathways and allow them to exert their physiological effects.

By attaching to VEGF receptors and ligands, VEGF, for example, can trigger angiogenesis. The effects of vascular endothelial growth factor (VEGF), as well as acidic and basic fibroblast growth factors (FGF1/2), can be employed to investigate the induction and progression of angiogenesis at various phases of tumour development. VEGF binds to its receptor (VEGFR) and ligands on the surface of ECs. It causes dimerization, autophosphorylation, and activation of the downstream signalling cascade after binding to and activating the transmembrane tyrosine kinase receptors on the cell's surface [94–96]. Tube development and sprouting follow EC survival, proliferation, migration, and apoptosis avoidance through several cascade phases. Over time, this process results in the development of a complex network of new blood vessels. Vasodilation and vascular permeability, a key feature of tissue inflammation and the tumour microenvironment, are also induced by VEGF [97–103].

The activity of the ECs outlined above is caused by an increase in pro-angiogenic factors such as VEGF and proteolytic enzymes, as well as a decrease in anti-angiogenic factors. Finally, a capillary network is successfully established, supplying enough nutrition and oxygen to the growing tumour. Taking advantage of this new vascular bed, the tumour cell may reach the systemic circulation and induce distant metastases. As a result, the number of metastasis sites is proportional to the amount of cancer cells that enter the circulation at the outset [104–111].

Angiogenic inducers have been implicated in the regulating process of angiogenesis in malignancies since their discovery a decade ago. Anti-angiogenic treatment decreases tumour vascular growth by interfering with VEGF and VEGFR intracellular signalling [112–116].

Angiogenesis was originally linked to cancer, arthritis, and psoriasis. However, the impact it has on a variety of other disorders has been documented. Tumours are innately primed for successful angiogenic development due to their nature and composition. An active vascular system is made up of adipose tissue that is encased in stromal cells and serves as a scaffold for the tumour's vascular system to emerge [117–119].

Brown adipose tissue (made up of cells with numerous mitochondria) promotes tumour growth by supplying a steady supply of oxygen and nutrients, whereas white adipose tissue promotes the formation and progression of breast cancer in a mouse model. Both types of adipose tissues, which have been associated to breast cancer, produce angiogenic factors such as VEGF A, B, and C, basic fibroblast growth factor (bFGF)/FGF-2, matrix metalloproteinases (MMPs), and IL-8. This aberrant blood vessel creation has been linked to cardiovascular illness, cancer, blindness, and diabetic ulcers [120–122].

2.5 Non-angiogenic functions of VEGF in breast cancer

VEGF increases the formation of new blood vessels and lymphatics, as well as increasing vascular permeability, and has a variety of tumour-related effects. The importance of VEGF in vascular and lymphangiogenesis has dominated research in breast and other cancers [123]. The importance of VEGF in cancer behaviour cannot be overstated. The presence of hypoxic patches in most malignancies, on the other hand, implies that VEGF-induced angiogenesis is insufficient to alleviate hypoxia [124]. Hypoxia works as a strong selection pressure, allowing only the most aggressive and metastatic cells to thrive. Understanding the mechanisms that allow tumour cells to survive under hypoxia is therefore critical for interpreting cancer biology and developing therapeutic approaches [125, 126].

VEGF produced by tumour or stromal cells interacts to VEGF receptors on tumour cells, producing a signalling response that supports survival in the face of hypoxia and other apoptotic triggers, according to our and other labs' research [127]. This process, which most likely operates in tandem with p53 inactivation, provides self-sufficiency to tumour cells, making it simpler for them to form tumours and increasing the possibility that they will spread to other parts of the body [128, 129]. To put it another way, we believe that hypoxia favours cells that can signal VEGF, and that the most aggressive tumour cells (metastatic cells) are determined by their dependency on VEGF.

A side effect of VEGF signalling in breast cancer cells is that it can help them move and invade more easily.

3. Breast carcinoma cells and VEGF signalling

3.1 Survival signalling by autocrine VEGF

Tumour cells receive signals from various sources as a result of the complex microenvironment of solid tumours, and these signals alter the activity of other cells. However, it is becoming obvious that cancer cells can attain a certain level of self-sufficiency by creating autocrine signalling pathways that aid critical tasks such as growth, survival, and invasion [130] within this web of paracrine signalling. As tumours develop towards invasive and metastatic illness, autocrine pathways become more critical as the tumour's environment becomes increasingly hostile. As a result, autocrine signalling pathways are a major target for anti-tumour therapy. Our study on invasive breast carcinoma cell lines provided one of the first indications that VEGF may have autocrine functions in cancer [73, 131].

We discovered that a 50% reduction in VEGF expression resulted in a considerable increase in apoptosis, even in the presence of 10% serum, when we utilised an anti-sense oligonucleotide approach to limit VEGF expression. This evidence backs with the theory that these cells were selected in vivo because they rely on VEGF to survive [132]. The importance of VEGF in carcinoma and other cancer cell survival has now been validated by research from our lab and others.

Because it increased VEGF expression in invasive breast cancer cell lines, hypoxia inhibited apoptosis caused by serum deprivation. The mechanism by which autocrine VEGF maintains the survival of breast carcinoma cells appears to involve constitutive activation of the PI3-kinase pathway, as evidenced by the findings that reducing VEGF expression results in a significant decrease in PI3-kinase basal activity, hypoxia stimulates Akt activity, and inhibition of PI3-kinase induces apoptosis [133]. According to previous studies, VEGF inhibits apoptosis in breast cancer cells via upregulating the anti-apoptotic protein Bcl-2.

3.2 The role of VEGF in breast carcinoma migration and invasion

Carcinoma cells acquire the ability to migrate and infiltrate tissues as a result of malignant transformation and development. Although chemoattractant gradients may enhance carcinoma migration and invasion, it has been established that cells' ability to form autocrine signalling pathways might boost their sensitivity to external stimuli [134]. Depleting VEGF expression in the presence of caspase inhibitors, which prevent apoptosis caused by VEGF expression loss, allowed us to find a role for autocrine VEGF in the migration and invasion of breast cancer cells towards chemokines. The capacity of breast cancer cells to migrate and invade in response to chemotactic stimuli is considerably diminished in such circumstances.

One mechanism for VEGF's involvement in these events is its ability to alter the expression of the chemokine receptor CXCR4 [135]. This finding is significant for breast cancer growth since stromal-derived factor-1, the receptor's ligand, is abundant in tumour stroma as well as organs such as the lymph and lung, which are the primary targets of invasive breast carcinoma cells, and CXCR4 inhibitors impede metastasis [136].

In addition to its survival benefits, VEGF autocrine signalling may contribute to tumour growth by boosting chemokine receptor expression and allowing tumour cells to migrate towards chemokine gradients [137].

3.3 Perspective

The revelation that breast cancer cells produce VEGF receptors is significant, but further research is needed to understand how these receptors are expressed as a result of transformation and progression, including EMT, and the mechanisms through which these receptors regulate tumour cell behaviour. Despite having inherent signalling capabilities, little is known about how NP-1 enhances VEGF165 signalling on breast cancer cells. In endothelial cells, it appears to work with either VEGFR1 or VEGFR2, although this has yet to be validated in breast cancer cells.

Another hypothesis is that NP-1 transmits NP-1 signals in neurons via interacting with non-VEGF receptors in cancer cells, such as plexins. Our findings reveal that plexin A1 is expressed in breast cancer cells and can affect cell motility. The study of plexin involvement in NP-1 signalling will require a much more in-depth understanding of plexin expression and function in breast and other cancers. In addition, more exact data on the location and relative expression of NP-1 in the mammary gland and human breast malignancies is needed.

VEGF-C and VEGF-D, for example, have been linked to angiogenesis and lymphangiogenesis in breast tumours. It's critical to figure out whether these VEGFs have a paracrine or autocrine effect on breast cancer cells. Some data suggests that breast cancer cells can respond to VEGF-D autocrinely, although additional research is needed to confirm this.

Author details

Pooja G. Singh[1], Kanthesh M. Basalingappa[2*], T.S. Gopenath[3] and B.V. Sushma[1]

1 Department of Nutrition and Dietetics, School of Life Sciences, JSS AHER, Mysuru, India

2 Division of Molecular Biology, School of Life Sciences, JSS AHER, Mysuru, India

3 Department of Biotechnology and Bioinformatics, School of Life Sciences, JSS AHER, Mysuru, India

*Address all correspondence to: kantheshmb@jssuni.edu.in

References

[1] Folkman J. Tumor angiogenesis theraperutic implications. The New England Journal of Medicine. 1971;**285**:1182-1186

[2] Muthukkaruppan VR, Kubai L, Auerbach R. Tumor-induced neovascularization in the mouse eye. Journal of the National Cancer Institute. 1982;**69**:699-708

[3] Holmgren L, O'Reilly MS, Folkman J. Dormancy of micrometastases: Balance proliferation and apoptosis in the presence of angiogenesis suppression. Nature Medicine. 1995;**1**:149-153

[4] Parangi S, O'Reilly M, Christofori G, et al. Angiogenesis therapy of transgenic mice impairs de novo tumor growth. Proceedings of the National Academy of Sciences of the United States of America. 1996;**93**:2002-2007

[5] Denekamp J. Angiogenesis, neovascular proliferation and vascular pathophysiology as targets for cancer therapy. The British Journal of Radiology. 1993;**66**:181-196

[6] Dameron KM, Volpert OV, Tainsky MA, et al. Control of angiogenesis in fibroblasts by p53 regulation of thorombospongin-1. Science. 1994;**265**:1582-1584

[7] Miller KD. Recent translational research: Antiangiogenic therapy for breast cancer: Where do we stand? Breast Cancer Research. 2004;**6**:128-132

[8] Kerbel RS. A cancer therapy resistant to resistance. Nature. 1997;**390**:335-336

[9] Folkman J. Angiogenesis in cancer, vascular, rheumatoid and other disease. Nature Medicine. 1995;**1**:27-31

[10] Engels K, Fox SB, Whitehouse RM, Gatter KC, Harris AL. Distinct angiogenic patterns are associated with high-grade in situ ductal carcinomas of the breast. The Journal of Pathology. 1997;**181**:207-212

[11] Gasparini G, Harris AL. Clinical importance of the determination of tumor angiogenesis in breast carcinoma: Much more than a new prognostic tool. Journal of Clinical Oncology. 1995;**13**:765-782

[12] Linderholm B, Lindh B, Tavelin B, Grankvist K, Henriksson R. p53 and vascular endothelial growth factor expression predicts outcome in 833 patients with primary breast carconoma. International Journal of Cancer. 2000;**89**:51-62

[13] Siourdsson H, Baldetorp B, Boro A, et al. Indicators of prognosis in node-negative breast cancer. The New England Journal of Medicine. 1990;**322**:1045-1053

[14] American Cancer Society. Available from: https://www.cancer.org/research/cancer-facts-statistics/breast-cancer-facts-figures.html

[15] DeSantis C, Ma J, Bryan L, Jemal A. Breast cancer statistics, 2013. CA Cancer Journal. 2014;**64**:52-62

[16] American Cancer Society. Breast Cancer Facts & Figures 2015-2016. Atlanta: American Cancer Society, Inc.; 2015

[17] Castañeda-Gill JM, Vishwanatha JK. Antiangiogenic mechanisms and factors in breast cancer treatment. Journal of Carcinogenesis. 2016;**15**:1

[18] Coelho AL, Gomes MP, Catarino RJ, et al. Angiogenesis in

NSCLC: Is vessel co-option the trunk that sustains the branches? Oncotarget. 2017;**8**:39795-39804

[19] Sim EK, Zhang L, Shim WS, Lim YL, Ge R. Therapeutic angiogenesis for coronary artery disease. Journal of Cardiac Surgery. 2002;**17**:350-354

[20] Risau W, Flamme I. Vasculogenesis. Annual Review of Cell and Developmental Biology. 1995;**11**:73-91

[21] Hanahan D, Weinberg RA. Weinberg, Hallmarks of cancer: The next generation. Cell. 2011;**144**:646-674

[22] Folkman J, Browder T, Palmblad J. Angiogenesis research: Guidelines for translation to clinical application. Thrombosis and Haemostasis. 2001;**86**:23-33

[23] Tannock IF. The relation between cell proliferation and the vascular system in a transplanted mouse mammary tumour. British Journal of Cancer. 1968;**22**:258-273

[24] Carmeliet P. Angiogenesis in life, disease and medicine. Nature. 2005;**438**:932-936

[25] Hanahan D, Folkman J. Patterns and emerging mechanisms of the angiogenic switch during tumorigenesis. Cell. 1996;**86**:353-364

[26] Grimm D, Wehland M, Pietsch J, et al. Drugs interfering with apoptosis in breast cancer. Current Pharmaceutical Design. 2011;**17**:272-283. DOI: 10.2174/138161211795049723

[27] Grimm D, Bauer J, Schönberger J. Blockade of neoangiogenesis, a new and promising technique to control the growth of malignant tumors and its metastases. Current Vascular Pharmacology. 2009;**7**:347-357

[28] Folkman J, Shing Y. Angiogenesis. The Journal of Biological Chemistry. 1992;**267**:10931-10934

[29] Folkman J. Tumour angiogenesis: Therapeutic implications. The New England Journal of Medicine. 1971;**285**:1182-1186

[30] Fong G, Rossant J, Gartsenstein M, et al. Role of the Flt-1 receptor tyrosine kinase in regulating the assembly of vascular endothelium. Nature. 1995;**376**:67-70

[31] Shalably F, Rossant J, Yamaguchi TP, et al. Failure of blood island formation and vasculogenesis in FLK-1 deficient mice. Nature. 1995;**376**:62-66

[32] Horak ER, Klenk N, Leek R, et al. Angiogenesis, assessed by platelet/EC adhesion molecule antibodies, as indicator of node metastases and survival in breast cancer. Lancet. 1992;**340**:1120-1124

[33] Vartanian RK, Weidner N. Correlation of intratumoral EC proliferation with microvessel density (tumor angiogenesis) and tumor cell proliferation in breast carcinoma. The American Journal of Pathology. 1994;**144**:1188-1194

[34] Weidner N, Semple JP, Welch WR, et al. Tumor angiogenesis and metastasis– correlation in invasive breast carcinoma. The New England Journal of Medicine. 1991;**324**:1-8

[35] Linderholm B, Tavelin B, Grankvist K, et al. Does vascular endothelial growth factor (VEGF) predict local relapse and survival in radiotherapytreated node-negative breast cancer? British Journal of Cancer. 1999;**81**:727-732

[36] George ML, Tutton MG, Janssen F, et al. VEGF-A, VEGF-C, and VEGF-D in colorectal cancer progression. Neoplasia. 2001;**3**:420-427

[37] Holmgren L, O'Reilly MS, Folkman J. Dormancy of micrometastases: Balanced proliferation and apoptosis in the presence of angiogenesis suppression. Nature Medicine. 1995;**1**:149-153

[38] Linderholm BK, Hellborg H, Johansson U, et al. Significantly higher levels of vascular endothelial growth factor (VEGF) and shorter survival times for patients with primary operable triple-negative breast cancer. Annals of Oncology. 2009;**20**:1639-1646

[39] FDA Approval for Bevacizumab. 2015. Available from: http://www.cancer.gov/cancertopics/druginfo/fda-bevacizumab

[40] Tarallo V, De Falco S. The vascular endothelial growth factors and receptors family: Up to now the only target for anti-angiogenesis therapy. The International Journal of Biochemistry & Cell Biology. 2015;**64**:185-189

[41] Bellou S, Pentheroudakis G, Murphy C, et al. Anti-angiogenesis in cancer therapy: Hercules and Hydra. Cancer Letters. 2013;**338**:219-228

[42] Ivy SP, Wick JY, Kaufman BM. An overview of small-molecule inhibitors of VEGFR signaling. Nature Reviews: Clinical Oncology. 2009;**6**:569-579

[43] Miles DW, Chan A, Dirix LY, et al. Phase III study of bevacizumab plus docetaxel compared with placebo plus docetaxel for the first-line treatment of human epidermal growth factor receptor 2-negative metastatic breast cancer. Journal of Clinical Oncology. 2010;**28**:3239-3247

[44] Robert NJ, Dieras V, Glaspy J, et al. RIBBON-1: Randomized, double-blind, placebo-controlled, phase III trial of chemotherapy with or without bevacizumab for first-line treatment of human epidermal growth factor receptor 2-negative, locally recurrent or metastatic breast cancer. Journal of Clinical Oncology. 2011;**29**:1252-1260

[45] Elcieri BP, Cheresh DA. Adhesion events in angiogenesis. Current Opinion in Cell Biology. 2001;**13**:563-568

[46] Kubota Y, Kleinman HK, Martin GR, Lawley TJ. Role of laminin and basement membrane in the morphological differentiation of human endothelial cells into capillary-like structures. The Journal of Cell Biology. 1988;**107**:1589-1596

[47] Wang GL, Jiang BH, Rue EA, Semenza GL. Hypoxia inducible factor is a basic helix-loop-helix PAS heterodimer regulated by cellular oxygen tension. Proceedings of the National Academy of Science USA. 1995;**92**:5510-5514

[48] Masson N, Willam C, Maxwell PH, Pugh CW, Ratcliffe PJ. Independent function of two destruction domains in hypoxiainducible factor-alpha chains activated by prolyl hydroxylation. The EMBO Journal. 2001;**20**:5197-5206

[49] Maxwell PH, Dachs GU, Gleadle JM, Nicholls LG, Harris AL, Stratford IJ, et al. Hypoxia-inducible factor-1 modulates gene expression in solid tumors and influences both angiogenesis and tumor growth. Proceedings of the National Academy of Science USA. 1997;**94**:8104-8109

[50] Carmeliet P, Dor Y, Herbert JM, Fukumura D, Brusselmans K, Dewerchin M, et al. Role of Hif-1alpha in hypoxia-mediated apoptosis, cell proliferation and tumour angiogenesis. Nature. 1998;**394**:485-490

[51] Bos R, Zhong H, Hanrahan CF, Mommers EC, Semenza GL, Pinedo HM, et al. Levels of hypoxia-inducible factor-1 alpha during breast carcinogenesis. Journal of the National Cancer Institute. 2001;**93**:309-314. DOI: 10.1093/jnci/93.4.309

[52] Forsythe JA, Jiang BH, Iyer NV, Agani F, Leung SW, Koos RD, et al. Activation of vascular endothelial growth factor gene transcription by hypoxia-inducible factor 1. Molecular and Cellular Biology. 1996;**16**:4604-4613

[53] Gerber HP, Condorelli F, Park J, Ferrara N. Differential transcriptional regulation of the two vascular endothelial growth factor receptor genes. Flt-1, but not Flk-1/KDR, is up-regulated by hypoxia. The Journal of Biological Chemistry. 1997;**272**:23659-23667

[54] Olofsson B, Jeltsch M, Eriksson U, Alitalo K. Current biology of Vegf-B and Vegf-C. Current Opinion in Biotechnology. 1999;**10**:528-535

[55] Brown LF, Guidi AJ, Schnitt SJ, Van De Water L, Iruela-Arispe ML, Yeo TK, et al. Vascular stroma formation in carcinoma in situ, invasive carcinoma, and metastatic carcinoma of the breast. Clinical Cancer Research. 1999;**5**:1041-1056

[56] Hattori K, Heissig B, Wu Y, Dias S, Tejada R, Ferris B, et al. Placental growth factor reconstitutes hematopoiesis by recruiting VEGFR1(+) stem cells from bonemarrow microenvironment. Nature Medicine. 2002;**8**:841-849

[57] Luttun A, Tjwa M, Moons L, Wu Y, Angelillo-Scherrer A, Liao F, et al. Revascularization of ischemic tissues by PlGF treatment, and inhibition of tumor angiogenesis, arthritis and atherosclerosis by anti-Flt1. Nature Medicine. 2002;**8**:831-840

[58] Dvorak HF, Sioussat TM, Brown LF, Berse B, Nagy JA, Sotrel A, et al. Distribution of vascular permeability factor (vascular endothelial growth factor) in tumors: Concentration in tumor blood vessels. The Journal of Experimental Medicine. 1991;**174**:1275-1278. DOI: 10.1084/jem.174.5.1275

[59] Hashizume H, Baluk P, Morikawa S, McLean JW, Thurston G, Roberge S, et al. Openings between defective endothelial cells explain tumor vessel leakiness. The American Journal of Pathology. 2000;**156**:1363-1380. DOI: 10.1016/s0002-9440(10)65006-7

[60] Guidi AJ, Schnitt SJ, Fischer L, Tognazzi K, Harris JR, Dvorak HF, et al. Vascular permeability factor (vascular endothelial growth factor) expression and angiogenesis in patients with ductal carcinoma in situ of the breast. Cancer. 1997;**80**:1945-1953

[61] Greb RR, Maier I, Wallwiener D, Kiesel L. Vascular endothelial growth factor a (Vegf-a) mRNA expression levels decrease after menopause in normal breast tissue but not in breast cancer lesions. British Journal of Cancer. 1999;**81**:225-231

[62] Losordo DW, Isner JM. Estrogen and angiogenesis: A review. Arteriosclerosis, Thrombosis, and Vascular Biology. 2001;**21**:6-12

[63] Hyder SM, Murthy L, Stancel GM. Progestin regulation of vascular endothelial growth factor in human breast cancer cells. Cancer Research. 1998;**58**:392-395

[64] Ruohola JK, Valve EM, Karkkainen MJ, Joukov V, Alitalo K, Harkonen PL. Vascular endothelial growth factors are differentially regulated by steroid hormones and

antiestrogens in breast cancer cells. Molecular and Cellular Endocrinology. 1999;**149**:29-40

[65] Buteau-Lozano H, Ancelin M, Lardeux B, Milanini J, PerrotApplanat M. Transcriptional regulation of vascular endothelial growth factor by estradiol and tamoxifen in breast cancer cells: A complex interplay between estrogen receptors alpha and beta. Cancer Research. 2002;**62**:4977-4984

[66] Takei H, Lee ES, Jordan CV. In vitro regulation of vascular endothelial growth factor by estrogens and antiestrogens in estrogen-receptor positive breast cancer. Breast Cancer. 2002;**9**:39-42

[67] Scorilas A, Karameris A, ArnogiannakiN,ArdavanisA,BassilopoulosP, Trangas T, et al. Overexpression of matrix-metalloproteinase-9 in human breast cancer: A potential favourable indicator in node-negative patients. British Journal of Cancer. 2001;**84**:1488-1496

[68] Bergers G, Brekken R, McMahon G, Vu TH, Itoh T, Tamaki K, et al. Matrix metalloproteinase-9 triggers the angiogenic switch during carcinogenesis. Nature Cell Biology. 2000;**2**:737-744

[69] Bagheri-Yarmand R, Vadlamudi RK, Wang RA, Mendelsohn J, Kumar R. Vascular endothelial growth factor up-regulation via p21-activated kinase-1 signaling regulates heregulin-beta1- mediated angiogenesis. The Journal of Biological Chemistry. 2000;**275**:39451-39457

[70] Yen L, You XL, Al Moustafa AE, Batist G, Hynes NE, Mader S, et al. Heregulin selectively upregulates vascular endothelial growth factor secretion in cancer cells and stimulates angiogenesis. Oncogene. 2000;**19**:3460-3469

[71] Petit AM, Rak J, Hung MC, Rockwell P, Goldstein N, Fendly B, et al. Neutralizing antibodies against epidermal growth factor and ErbB-2/neu receptor tyrosine kinases down-regulate vascular endothelial growth factor production by tumor cells in vitro and in vivo: Angiogenic implications for signal transduction therapy of solid tumors. The American Journal of Pathology. 1997;**151**:1523-1530

[72] Laughner E, Taghavi P, Chiles K, Mahon PC, Semenza GL. HER2 (neu) signaling increases the rate of hypoxia-inducible factor 1alpha (HIF-1alpha) synthesis: Novel mechanism for HIF-1- mediated vascular endothelial growth factor expression. Molecular and Cellular Biology. 2001;**21**:3995-4004

[73] Chung J, Bachelder RE, Lipscomb EA, Shaw LM, Mercurio AM. Integrin (alpha 6 beta 4) regulation of eIF-4E activity and VEGF translation: A survival mechanism for carcinoma cells. The Journal of Cell Biology. 2002;**158**:165-174

[74] Edel MJ, Harvey JM, Papadimitriou JM. Comparison of vascularity and angiogenesis in primary invasive mammary carcinomas and in their respective axillary lymph node metastases. Clinical & Experimental Metastasis. 2000;**18**:695-702

[75] Monsky WL, Mouta Carreira C, Tsuzuki Y, Gohongi T, Fukumura D, Jain RK. Role of host microenvironment in angiogenesis and microvascular functions in human breast cancer xenografts: Mammary fat pad versus cranial tumors. Clinical Cancer Research. 2002;**8**:1008-1013

[76] Lee JC, Kim DC, Gee MS, Saunders HM, Sehgal CM, Feldman MD,

et al. Interleukin-12 inhibits angiogenesis and growth of transplanted but not in situ mouse mammary tumor virus-induced mammary carcinomas. Cancer Research. 2002;**62**:747-755

[77] Animal models to study mammary gland development, physiology and tumorigenesis. Available from: http://mammary.nih.gov/models/index.html

[78] Fidler I, Ellis L. The implications of angiogenesis for the biology and therapy of cancer metastasis. Cell. 1994;**79**:185-188

[79] Papetti M, Herman IM. Mechanisms of normal and tumor-derived angiogenesis. American Journal of Physiology: Cell Physiology. 2002;**282**:947-970

[80] Liekens S, De Clercq E, Neyts J. Angiogenesis: Regulators and clinical applications. Biochemical Pharmacology. 2001;**61**:253-270

[81] Maj E, Papiernik D, Wietrzyk J. Antiangiogenic cancer treatment: The great discovery and greater complexity (review). International Journal of Oncology. 2016;**49**:1773-1784

[82] Singh RK, Gutman M, Bucana CD, et al. Sequential development of an angiogenic phenotype by human fibroblasts progressing to tumorigenicity. Proceedings of the National Academy of Science USA. 1995;**92**:4562-4566

[83] Kandel J, Bossy-Wetzel E, Radvanyi F, et al. Neovascularization is associated with a switch to the export of bFGF in the multistep development of fibrosarcoma. Cell. 1991;**66**:1095-1104

[84] Folkman J, Hanahan D. Switch to the angiogenic phenotype during tumorigenesis. Princess Takamatsu Symposia. 1991;**22**:339-347

[85] Good DJ, Polverini PJ, Rastinejad F, et al. A tumor suppressor–dependent inhibitor of angiogenesis is immunologically and functionally indistinguishable from a fragment of thrombospondin. Proceedings of the National Academy of Science USA. 1990;**87**:6624-6628

[86] Rastinejad F, Polverini PJ, Bouck NP. Regulation of the activity of a new inhibitor of angiogenesis by a cancer suppressor gene. Cell. 1989;**56**:345-355

[87] Tang N, Wang L, Esko J, et al. Loss of HIF-1alpha in endothelial cells disrupts a hypoxia-driven VEGF autocrine loop necessary for tumorigenesis. Cancer Cell. 2004;**6**:485-495

[88] Harris AL. Hypoxia—A key regulatory factor in tumour growth. Nature Reviews: Cancer. 2002;**2**:38-47. DOI: 10.1038/nrc704

[89] Semenza GL. HIF-1 and tumor progression: Pathophysiology and therapeutics. Trends in Molecular Medicine. 2002;**8**:S62-S67

[90] Zhong H, De Marzo AM, Laughner E, et al. Overexpression of hypoxia-inducible factor 1alpha in common human cancers and their metastases. Cancer Research. 1999;**59**:5830-5835

[91] Bertout JA, Patel SA, Simon MC. The impact of O_2 availability on human cancer. Nature Reviews: Cancer. 2008;**8**:967-975

[92] Mazure NM, Brahimi-Horn MC, Berta MA, Benizri E, Bilton RL, Dayan F, et al. HIF-1: Master and commander of the hypoxic world: A pharmacological approach to its regulation by siRNAs. Biochemical Pharmacology. 2004;**68**:971-980

[93] Semenza GL. Targeting HIF-1 for cancer therapy. Nature Reviews: Cancer. 2003;**3**:721-732

[94] Claesson-Welsh L, Welsh MJ. VEGFA and tumour angiogenesis. Internal Medicine. 2013;**273**:114-127

[95] Mendelsohn J, Howley P, Israel M, Liotta L. The Molecular Basis of Cancer. Philadelphia: W. B. Saunders; 1995. pp. 206-232

[96] Senger DR, Galli SJ, Dvorak AM, et al. Tumor cells secrete a vascular permeability factor that promotes accumulation of ascites fluid. Science. 1983;**219**:983-985

[97] Felmeden DC, Blann AD, Lip GYH. Angiogenesis: Basic pathophysiology and implications for disease. European Heart Journal. 2003;**24**:586-603

[98] Leung DW, Cachianes G, Kuang WJ, Goeddel DV, Ferrara N. Vascular endothelial growth factor is a secreted angiogenic mitogen. Science. 1989;**246**:1306-1309

[99] Keck PJ, Hauser SD, Krivi G, et al. Vascular permeability factor, an endothelial cell mitogen related to PDGF. Science. 1989;**246**:1309-1312

[100] Connolly DT, Heuvelman DM, Nelson R, et al. Tumor vascular permeability factor stimulates endothelial cell growth and angiogenesis. The Journal of Clinical Investigation. 1989;**84**:1470-1478

[101] Tischer E, Gospodarowicz D, Mitchell R, et al. Vascular endothelial growth factor: A new member of the platelet derived growth factor gene family. Biochemical and Biophysical Research. 1989;**165**:1198-1206

[102] Ferrara N, Houck K, Jakeman L, et al. Molecular and biological properties of vascular endothelial growth factor family of protein. Endocrine Reviews. 1992;**13**:18-32

[103] Kristensen TB, Knutsson MLT, Wehland M, et al. Anti-vascular endothelial growth factor therapy in breast cancer. International Journal of Molecular Sciences. 2014;**15**:23024-23041

[104] Maxwell PH, Wiesener MS, Chang G-W, et al. The tumour suppressor protein VHL targets hypoxia-inducible factors for oxygen-dependent proteolysis. Nature. 1999;**399**:271-275

[105] Park JE, Keller GA, Ferrara N. The vascular endothelial growth factor (VEGF) isoforms: Differential deposition into the subepithelial extracellular matrix and bioactivity of extracellular matrix-bound VEGF. Molecular Biology of the Cell. 1993;**4**:1317-1326

[106] Li B, Leung DW, et al. The vascular endothelial growth factor family: Identification of a fourth molecular species and characterization of alternative splicing of RNA. Molecular Endocrinology. 1991;**5**:1806-1814

[107] Ferrara N, Gerber HP, LeCouter J. The biology of VEGF and its receptors. Nature Medicine. 2003;**9**:669-676

[108] Olsson AK, Dimberg A, Kreuger J, Claesson-Welsh L. VEGF receptor signalling—In control of vascular function. Nature Reviews: Molecular Cell Biology. 2006;**7**:359-371

[109] Bottaro DP, Liotta LA. Cancer: Out of air is not out of action. Nature. 2003;**423**:593-595

[110] Zhao Y, Adjei AA. Targeting angiogenesis in cancer therapy: Moving beyond vascular endothelial growth factor. The Oncologist. 2015;**20**:660-673

[111] Koch S, Claesson-Welsh L. Signal transduction by vascular endothelial growth factor receptors. Cold Spring

Harbor Perspectives in Medicine. July 2012;**2**(7):a006502

[112] Pepper MS, Ferrara N, Orci L, Montesano R. Potent synergism between vascular endothelial growth factor and basic fibroblast growth factor in the induction of angiogenesis in vitro. Biochemical and Biophysical Research Communications. 1992;**189**:824-831

[113] Korpanty G, Smyth E, Carney DN. Update on anti-angiogenic therapy in non-small cell lung cancer: Are we making progress? Journal of Thoracic Disease. 2011;**3**:19-29

[114] Heusschen R, van Gink M, Griffioen AW, Thijssen VL. MicroRNAs in the tumor endothelium: Novel controls on the angioregulatory switchboard. Biochimica et Biophysica Acta. 2010;**1805**:87-96

[115] Wahl ML, Moser TL, Pizzo SV. Angiostatin and anti-angiogenic therapy in human disease. Recent Progress in Hormone Research. 2004;**59**:73-104

[116] Lee SH, Jeung IC, Park TW, et al. Extension of the in vivo half-life of endostatin and its improved anti-tumor activities upon fusion to a humanized antibody against tumor-associated glycoprotein 72 in a mouse model of human colorectal carcinoma. Oncotarget. 2015;**6**:7182-7194

[117] Caporali A, Emanueli C. MicroRNA regulation in angiogenesis. Vascular Pharmacology. 2011;**55**:79-86

[118] Butler TP, Gullino PM. Quantitation of cell shedding into efferent blood of mammary adenocarcinoma. Cancer Research. 1975;**35**:512-516

[119] Bouck N, Stellmach V, Hsu S. How tumors become angiogenic. Advances in Cancer Research. 1996;**69**:135-174

[120] Folkman J. Tumor angiogenesis. In: The Molecular Basis of Cancer. 1995. Available from: https://www.nature.com/articles/nm0195-27#auth-Judah-Folkman. DOI: 10.1016/s0065-230x(08)60946-x

[121] Folkman J. Clinical applications of research on angiogenesis. The New England Journal of Medicine. 1995;**333**:1757-1763. DOI: 10.1056/NEJM199512283332608

[122] Wehland M, Bauer J, Magnusson NE, et al. Biomarkers for anti-angiogenic therapy in cancer. International Journal of Molecular Sciences. 2013;**14**:9338-9364. DOI: 10.3390%2Fijms14059338

[123] Dvorak HF, Nagy JA, Feng D, Brown LF, Dvorak AM. Vascular permeability factor/vascular endothelial growth factor and the significance of microvascular hyperpermeability in angiogenesis. Current Topics in Microbiology and Immunology. 1999;**237**:97-132

[124] Hockel M, Vaupel P. Tumor hypoxia: Definitions and current clinical, biologic, and molecular aspects. Journal of the National Cancer Institute. 2001;**93**:266-276

[125] Bachelder RE, Crago A, Chung J, Wendt MA, Shaw LM, Robinson G, et al. Vascular endothelial growth factor is an autocrine survival factor for neuropilin-expressing breast carcinoma cells. Cancer Research. 2001;**61**:5736-5740

[126] Harmey JH, Bouchier-Hayes D. Vascular endothelial growth factor (VEGF), a survival factor for tumour cells: Implications for anti-angiogenic therapy. BioEssays. 2002;**24**:280-283

[127] Bates RC, Goldsmith JD, Bachelder RE, Brown C, Shibuya M,

Oettgen P, et al. Flt-1 (VEGFR-1)-dependent survival characterizes the epithelial-mesenchymal transition of colonic organoids. Current Biology. 2003;**13**:1721-1727

[128] Sharieff W. Bevacizumab in colorectal cancer. New England Journal of Medicine. 2004;**351**:1690-1691

[129] Brusselmans K, Bono F, Collen D, Herbert JM, Carmeliet P, Dewerchin M. A novel role for vascular endothelial growth factor as an autocrine survival factor for embryonic stem cells during hypoxia. The Journal of Biological Chemistry. 2005;**280**:3493-3499

[130] Hanahan D, Weinberg RA. The hallmarks of cancer. Cell. 2000;**100**:57-70

[131] Masood R, Cai J, Zheng T, Smith DL, Hinton DR, Gill PS. Vascular endothelial growth factor (VEGF) is an autocrine growth factor for VEGF receptor-positive human tumors. Blood. 2001;**98**:1904-1913

[132] Dias S, Hattori K, Heissig B, Zhu Z, Wu Y, Witte L, et al. Inhibition of both paracrine and autocrine VEGF/ VEGFR-2 signaling pathways is essential to induce long-term remission of xenotransplanted human leukemias. Proceedings of the National Academy of Science USA. 2001;**98**:10857-10862

[133] Bachelder RE, Wendt MA, Mercurio AM. Vascular endothelial growth factor promotes breast carcinoma invasion in an autocrine manner by regulating the chemokine receptor CXCR4. Cancer Research. 2002;**62**:7203-7206

[134] Shvartsman SY, Hagan MP, Yacoub A, Dent P, Wiley HS, Lauffenburger DA. Autocrine loops with positive feedback enable context-dependent cell signaling. American Journal of Physiology: Cell Physiology. 2002;**282**:C545-C559

[135] Muller A, Homey B, Soto H, Ge N, Catron D, Buchanan ME, et al. Involvement of chemokine receptors in breast cancer metastasis. Nature. 2001;**410**:50-56

[136] Luo Y, Raible D, Raper JA. Collapsin: A protein in brain that induces the collapse and paralysis of neuronal growth cones. Cell. 1993;**75**:217-227

[137] Bachelder RE, Lipscomb EA, Lin X, Wendt MA, Chadborn NH, Eickholt BJ, et al. Competing autocrine pathways involving alternative neuropilin-1 ligands regulate chemotaxis of carcinoma cells. Cancer Research. 2003;**63**:5230-5233

Chapter 2

Tumor Angiogenesis in Pituitary Adenoma

Daizo Yoshida and Akira Teramoto

Abstract

The role of angiogenesis in pituitary tumor development used to be questioned, since pituitary tumors have been usually found to be less vascularized than the normal pituitary tissue. Nevertheless, a significantly higher degree of vasculature has been shown in invasive or macropituitary prolactinomas when compared to noninvasive and microprolactinomas. We should know VEGF was found firstly in pituitary anterior lobe, then tumor angiogenesis must occur. Meanwhile the vascular arrangement raised by VEGF is irregular, that sometimes lead to pituitary apoplexy. In this chapter, hypoxia inducible factors (HIF), transcription factors regulating expression of several genes related to oxygen homeostasis are in response to hypoxic stress. We focus on tumor angiogenesis regulated by the signaling cascade in tumor angiogenesis in pituitary tumor.

Keywords: hypoxia inducible factors, tumor angiogenesis, pituitary adenoma

1. Introduction

Hypoxia is critical for the life. Autonomic nerves system responds to the hypoxia regulating circulatory and respiratory organs to ensure adequate oxygen delivery. Separately, cellular responses to hypoxia are mainly regulated by the activation of transcription factors called hypoxia-inducible factors (HIFs). HIFs affect hypoxia and stress response signaling pathways that influence development, metabolism, inflammation, and circulatory and respiratory physiology [1–5]. Hypoxia-inducible factors are also associated with many diseases in the circulatory system, mainly via VEGF. Copper is a co-factor of bFGF, accumulated in malignant glioma, the chelation inhibits glioma growth and angiogenesis in murine model. HIF pathways are triggered by hypoxia. The hypoxia regulates both in the cell signal level and in the circulatory and respiratory system by autonomic nerves. Hence, compromised response to ischemia is crucial. Inhibition of angiogenesis by reducing the HIF pathway can be a rational method in patients with ischemic diseases. Investigation regarding hypoxia mediated by intracellular signaling have been emerged as new targets focusing on the related genes or protein delivery to stabilize HIFs, but not yet accomplished. Oxygen tension is markedly below physiological levels in solid tumors also in pituitary adenoma. In fact, solid tumors contain severely hypoxic regions, in which pO_2 values are <10 mmHg [6, 7]. Tumor vessels raised by VEGF are regularly lacking tight junction, we consider that it leads pituitary apoplexy, hemorrhagic infarction.

In this chapter, we focus on the current understanding of the relationship between HIFs and pituitary adenoma in tumor angiogenesis.

2. Discussion

Endocan is known as endothelial cell-specific molecule-1 (ESM-1) that has a 50 kDa polypeptide with a single dermatan sulfate [8, 9]. After secreted from endothelial cell, endocan interacts between leukocyte function-associated antigen-1 (LFA-1) and intercellular adhesion molecule-1 (ICAM-1). Recent studies have shown that endocan mRNA expression in endothelial cells is specific to several angiogenic factors and cytokine, such as VEGF and TNF. Herein, function of endocan has been emerged in tumor hypoxia context. Endocan overexpress stimulates tumor progression in mouse models of human tumor xenografts. Anyway, these studies demonstrated that endocan can be a biomarker of tumor progression, and a potentially therapeutic target for cancer. Despite general immunotherapeutic therapy to cancer is not satisfactory, antibodies against endocan be still promising cancer treatment. Both plasma endocan and VEGF-A levels are elevated in patients with invasive tumor. Cornellius showed that, pituitary adenoma cells expressed endocan, though it was not observed in all normal pituitary [10]. Microvessels revealed significantly greater mean vessel areas in subgroups of tumors with endothelial endocan expression. Thus, endocan in endothelial cells may be a relevant marker of aggressiveness in pituitary tumors.

Two p53 binding sites are present in the promoter sequence of the gene encoding cathepsin D [11, 12] suggesting a direct relationship between cathepsin D and the induction of apoptosis. Cathepsin D is activated by an intracellular acid-dependent autoactivation mechanism. It has been reported that cathepsin D secreted by prostate carcinoma cells is responsible for the generation of angiostatin, an endogenous inhibitor of angiogenesis that is produced by the tumor-mediated proteolysis of plasminogen. Clinically, cathepsin D overexpression has been studied in several malignant tumor types [11] although most research has been focused on breast cancer, in which cathepsin D expression correlates with poor prognosis. Expression of cathepsin D is also significantly higher in malignant than in benign ovarian tumors [12]. In colon cancer cells, cathepsin D is upregulated by HIF 1α under hypoxic conditions, perhaps counteracting the effects of VEGF via angiostatin regulation [13]. Angiogenesis is a major mechanism by which oxygen supply is increased in tumors. Hypoxia has been found to regulate angiogenesis activators and may some- times downregulate angiogenesis inhibitors. In the mouse pituitary adenoma cell line GH4C, secretion of cathepsin D was inhibited under hypoxic conditions, suggesting that hypoxia acts directly on pituitary lactotrophs to inhibit PRL expression. In addition, cathepsin D can promote tumor invasiveness by acting as an autocrine growth factor within the pituitary to stimulate cell growth. The hormonal moiety in the hypoxia-responsive motif, however, has not yet been established.

In pituitary adenomas, regional oxygen saturation is lower than in normal pituitary lobes. VEGF and HIF-1α are also expressed in several pituitary adenomas; however, the role of HIF-1α and the relationship between HIF-1α and VEGF has been emerged Vidal et al. reported that HIF-1α was expressed in all types of pituitary adenoma and that the expression level in GH-producing pituitary adenomas and pituitary carcinomas was higher than in the other adenomas. We detected HIF-1α mRNA and protein in several pituitary adenoma types. Our statistical analysis confirmed earlier results that there was no significant correlation between HIF-1α expression and patient age, gender, and tumor size. GH-producing adenomas exhibited the highest, and ACTH-producing adenomas the lowest expression levels of HIF-1α; however, the difference was not statistically significant, possibly due to the small number of available samples. Our study confirmed earlier reports that VEGF was expressed in all types of pituitary adenoma [14, 15]. According to Lloyd et al., VEGF expression was high in GH-producing adenomas, corticotrophs, silent corticotrophs, silent subtype 3 tumors, non-oncocytic null-cell adenomas, and pituitary carcinomas [16]. However, between normal tissue and adenomas or tumors of different histotypes, there was no statistically significant difference with respect to VEGF expression. We also found no significant difference among the different adenoma types we examined.

We performed quantitative assessment of the expression of HIF-1α and VEGF in pituitary adenomas and examined the co-expression of HIF-1α and VEGF. Our results suggest that VEGF may be regulated not only by HIF-1α but by a different mechanism mediated by several cytokines and growth factors. In normal pituitary cells, pituitary adenylate cyclase-activating polypeptide (PACAP) and IL-6 can stimulate VEGF expression in vitro, whereas glucocorticoid has inhibitory action. In pituitary adenoma cells, VEGF expression was increased by TGF-α, PACAP, estradiol, IL-6, IGF-I, and pituitary tumor transforming gene (PTTG), and was inhibited by dexamethasone. Moreover, VEGF was co-localized with various pituitary hormones, suggesting that hypothalamic factors may play a role in the regulation of pituitary VEGF release. Therefore, the regulation of VEGF in pituitary tumors may not depend primarily on HIF-1α expression.

Our study also demonstrated that stromal cell-derived factor (SDF)-1 expression was positively correlated to microvascular density (MVD), strongly obvious in macroadenomas. Intensity for immunoreactivity for SDF-1 was not related. Given by these results we consider, abnormal blood vessels in the pituitary adenoma tissue may be not be able to supply the normal oxygen concentration like the normal vessels. Both SDF-1 mRNA and protein expression were firmly upregulated in hypoxia, and then regulate tumor angiogenesis in pituitary adenoma.

SDF-1 (CXCL12) is expressed both in embryo and cancer cell lines, and is an ELR-CXC chemokine that has angiogenic activity, role of the capillary-like formation stimulating human vascular endothelial cells also in pituitary adenoma [17]. Meanwhile CD34 is a cell-surface marker of hematopoietic stem cells (HSCs), mature vascular endothelial cells also express a receptor for SDF-1, CXCR4. CD34 cell migration is stimulate by CXCR4 via SDF-1 in vitro and could be a key factor for trafficking HSC between the peripheral blood and the bone marrow, named a homing effect. During embryogenesis, primitive blood vessels are shaped newly by the angioblasts aggregation, which is termed vasculogenesis.

In embryo, when the vasculogenesis starts mainly fibroblast growth factors (FGFs) cause some cells in the mesoderm differentiated into endothelial progenitors. SDF-1/CXCR4 axis has an initial role in all of hematopoiesis, vascular development, and cardiogenesis [18–20], whiles also in adults, homing of HSCs to the bone marrow and CD34 progenitor cell proliferation is regulated by SDF-1 [17]. Various organs, such as the liver, brain, and lymphoid organs widely expressed SDF-1. In particular, human ovarian cancer was firstly discuss to express high levels of SDF-1, and subsequently has been reported in glioblastoma.

Recently, several studies have focused on pituitary adenoma. Some showed that SDF-1 and its receptor, CXCR4, were expressed in rat pituitary adenomas, but they did not discuss the relationship between SDF-1 expression and angiogenesis [21–23]. Both prolactin and GH in the GH4C1 are regulated in cell proliferation and the release by CXCR4 activation, plausibly through complicated intracellular signals. However, discussion of exogenous SDF-1 has not yet clearly disclosed, because pituitary adenoma cells express CXCR4 but not SDF-1. Barbieri et al. analyzed the expression of both SDF-1 and CXCR4 in human pituitary adenomas, compared with normal hypophyses. They elucidated first the SDF-1 and CXCR4 expression in normal and adenomatous human pituitary and revealed that overexpression occurs in adenomas comparing normal-related pituitary cells, then indicating that this profile may contribute to the increasing proliferation [24].

Invasive pituitary adenoma has a complicated mechanism and interacts with the nerve-endocrine-immune network. It is affect DDR1 ligand combined with DDR1 can promote the DDR1 signaling pathway. DDR1 promotes MMP-2/9 expression, leading to ECM reconstruction and tumor invasion [25–27]. Cell apoptosis, change tumor cell invasiveness, and regulation of energy metabolism is mediated by hypoxic condition. Herein, discoidin domain receptor (DDR)-1 expression and its effect on pituitary adenoma under hypoxia still need further investigation. Our study confirmed that DDR1 mRNA and protein are elevated in primary pituitary adenoma cells along with hypoxia. Elevated DDR1 expression can regulated expression of MMP-2 and MMP-9 expression in supernatant, thereby promoting cell proliferation and invasion of pituitary adenoma. Nilotinib administration can diminish DDR1 expression and further reduce MMP-2 and -9 expression to reduce pituitary adenoma cells proliferation and invasion.

The above-mentioned factors have been discussed much few in pituitary adenoma. Cornelius et al. investigated that endocan, secreted by endothelial cells, associated with an aggressive behavior in pituitary tumors. The study by immunohistochemistry and reverse transcription polymerase chain reaction (RT-PCR) in patients operated for a pituitary adenoma, comparing normal post-mortem pituitaries. In normal pituitaries, endocan was never observed in vessels but was detectable in adenoma cells. In adenoma tissue, a significant relation between endocan immunoreactivity in endothelial cells and progression, tumor size, mitotic count, and p53 expression were demonstrated. The immunohistological study of endocan in endothelial cells therefore can be a new marker of aggressive behavior in pituitary tumors [28].

Cathepsin B expressed in invasive pituitary adenoma and is an important functional protein in apoptosis. One might hypothesize that shifting the balance between mediators of cell death could result in changes in pituitary tumor behavior [29].

Pituitary adenoma is considered to be benign, accounting 20% of intracranial tumors generally, that is the third most common intracranial tumor. But approximately 30% of pituitary adenomas are invasive. It can be said the already-established molecular mechanisms of the pituitary adenomas invasion, turning out mainly HIF-1α, pituitary tumor transforming gene, FGF-2, VEGF, and MMPs (mainly MMP-2, and MMP-9) are core signaling. These molecules have the ability to create a suitable microenvironment within the tumor. Together, they have a complicated interaction [30].

Nonfunctioning pituitary adenoma is sometime hard for surgery. However, there is no established conservative treatment. MicroRNA-134 (miR-134) may be promised that suppress tumor cell proliferation and invasion. Therefore, the effect of miR-134 on improving non-functioning pituitary tumor cells expansion is considered to be challenging. The molecular mechanism of the SDF-1α/miR-134/VEGFA axis is representative a novel mechanism in the pathogenesis of NF-PitNETs and may serve as a potential therapeutic target for the treatment of NF-PitNETs [31].

Study with flow cytometry show that the rates of CXCR4- and CXCL12-positive cells in invasive pituitary adenomas was significantly elevated in the cell suspensions than those in non-invasive pituitary adenomas. Immunohistochemical study unveiled that CXCR4 and CXCL12 staining index of the invasive pituitary adenomas were clearly higher than those of the non-invasive pituitary adenomas. Meanwhile, none of flow cytometry and immunohistochemistry could disclose significant difference between CD44 and CD147 expression, respectively. Then, CXCR4 and CXCL12 may potentially can be powerful biomarkers to detect early stage of pituitary adenomas [32].

Recently, Nilotinib has been highlighted to reduce DDR1 expression, decrease MMP-2 and MMP-9 expression, and inhibit pituitary adenoma cells proliferation and invasion [33].

Conclusively further investigations are required to elucidate the mechanisms underlying the invasiveness of pituitary adenoma-related phenomena is a new horizon in the field of neuro-oncology.

Conflict of interest

The authors declare no conflicts of interest.

Author details

Daizo Yoshida* and Akira Teramoto
Department of Neurological Surgery, Nippon Medical School, Yokyo Japan

*Address all correspondence to: dyoshida@nms.ac.jp

References

[1] Ke Q, Costa M. Hypoxia-inducible factor-1 (HIF-1). Molecular Pharmacology. 2006;**70**(5):1469-1480

[2] Fallah J, Rini BI. HIF inhibitors: Status of current clinical development. Current Oncology Reports. Jan 22 2019;**21**(1):6

[3] Albadari N, Deng S, Li W. The transcriptional factors HIF-1 and HIF-2 and their novel inhibitors in cancer therapy. Expert Opinion on Drug Discovery. Jul 2019;**14**(7):667-682

[4] Graham K, Unger E. Overcoming tumor hypoxia as a barrier to radiotherapy, chemotherapy and immunotherapy in cancer treatment. International Journal of Nanomedicine. Oct 2018;**13**:6049-6058

[5] Hsu TS, Lin YL, Wang YA, Mo ST, Chi PY, Lai AC, et al. HIF-2α is indispensable for regulatory T cell function. Nature Communications. Oct 6 2020;**11**(1):5005. DOI: 10.1038/s41467-020-18731-y

[6] Bhandari V, Hoey C, Liu LY, Lalonde E, Ray J, Livingstone J, et al. Molecular landmarks of tumor hypoxia across cancer types. Nature Genetics. Feb 2019;**51**(2):308-318

[7] De Freitas Caires N, Gaudet A, Portier L, Tsicopoulos A, Mathieu D, Lassalle P. Endocan, sepsis, pneumonia, and acute respiratory distress syndrome. Critical Care. Oct 26 2018;**22**(1):280

[8] Kuluöztürk M, İn E, İlhan N. Endocan as a marker of disease severity in pulmonary thromboembolism. The Clinical Respiratory Journal. Dec 2019;**13**(12):773-780

[9] Cornelius A, Cortet-Rudelli C, Assaker R, Kerdraon O, Gevaert M-H, Prévot V, et al. Endothelial expression of endocan is strongly associated with tumor progression in pituitary adenoma. Brain Pathology. 2012;**22**(6):757-764

[10] Minarowska A, Gacko M, Karwowska A, Minarowski Ł. Human cathepsin D. Folia Histochemica et Cytobiologica. 2008;**46**(1):23-38

[11] Kakimoto Y, Sasaki A, Niioka M, Kawabe N, Osawa M. Myocardial cathepsin D is downregulated in sudden cardiac death. PLoS One. Mar 16 2020;**15**(3). DOI: 10.1371/journal.pone.0230375

[12] Pranjol ZI, Whatmore JL. Cathepsin D in the tumor microenvironment of breast and ovarian cancers. Advances in Experimental Medicine and Biology. 2020;**1259**:1-16

[13] Basu S, Cheriyamundath S, Gavert N, Brabletz T, Haase G, Ben-Ze'ev A. Increased expression of cathepsin D is required for L1-mediated colon cancer progression. Oncotarget. Aug 27 2019;**10**(50):5217-5228

[14] Kim K, Yoshida D, Teramoto A. Expression of hypoxia-inducible factor 1alpha and vascular endothelial growth factor in pituitary adenomas. Endocrine Pathology. Summer 2005;**16**(2):115-121

[15] Yoshida D, Noha M, Watanabe K, Sugisaki Y, Teramoto A. Novel approach to analysis of in vitro tumor angiogenesis with a variable-pressure scanning electron microscope: Suppression by matrix metalloproteinase inhibitor SI-27. Tumor Pathology. 2001;**18**(2):89-100

[16] Vascular endothelial growth factor (VEGF) expression in human pituitary adenomas and carcinomas Ricardo V.

Lloyd, Bernd W. Scheithauer, Takao Kuroki, Sergio Vidal, Kalman Kovacs, Lucia Stefaneanu Endocrine Pathology. Autumn 1999;**10**(3):229-235

[17] Barbieri F, Bajetto A, Porcile C, Pattarozzi A, Schettini G, Florio T. Role of stromal cell-derived factor 1 (SDF1/CXCL12) in regulating anterior pituitary function. Journal of Molecular Endocrinology. Mar 2007;**38**(3):383-389

[18] Barbieri F, Bajetto A, Stumm R, Pattarozzi A, Porcile C, Zona G, et al. Overexpression of stromal cell-derived factor 1 and its receptor CXCR4 induces autocrine/paracrine cell proliferation in human pituitary adenomas. Clinical Cancer Research. Aug 15 2008;**14**(16):5651-5672

[19] Bajetto A, Barbieri F, Dorcaratto A, Barbero S, Daga A, Porcile C, et al. Expression of CXC chemokine receptors 1-5 and their ligands in human glioma tissues: Role of CXCR4 and SDF1 in glioma cell proliferation and migration. Neurochemistry International. Oct 2006;**49**(5):423-432

[20] Bajetto A, Bonavia R, Barbero S, Piccioli P, Costa A, Florio T, et al. Glial and neuronal cells express functional chemokine receptor CXCR4 and its natural ligand stromal cell-derived factor 1. Journal of Neurochemistry. Dec 1999;**73**(6):2348-2357

[21] Li S, Zhang Z, Xue J, Guo X, Liang S, Liu A. Effect of hypoxia on DDR1 expression in pituitary adenomas. Medical Science Monitor. Aug 19 2015;**21**:2433-2438

[22] Yoshida D, Teramoto A. Enhancement of pituitary adenoma cell invasion and adhesion is mediated by discoidin domain receptor-1. Journal of Neuro-Oncology. Mar 2007;**82**(1):29-40

[23] Hilton HN, Stanford PM, Harris J, Oakes SR, Kaplan W, Daly RJ, et al. KIBRA interacts with discoidin domain receptor 1 to modulate collagen-induced signalling. Biochimica et Biophysica Acta. Mar 2008;**1783**(3):383-389

[24] Porcile C, Bajetto A, Barbieri F, Barbero S, Bonavia R, Biglieri M, et al. Stromal cell-derived factor-1alpha (SDF-1alpha/CXCL12) stimulates ovarian cancer cell growth through the EGF receptor transactivation. Experimental Cell Research. Aug 15 2005;**308**(2):241-253

[25] Yang Q, Li X. Molecular network basis of invasive pituitary adenoma: A review. Frontiers in Endocrinology. Jan 24 2019;**10**:7

[26] Ruskyte K, Liutkevicienė R, Vilkeviciute A, Vaitkiene P, Valiulytė I, Glebauskiene B, et al. MMP-14 and TGFbeta-1 methylation in pituitary adenomas. Oncology Letters. Oct 2016;**12**(4):3013-3017

[27] Gupta P, Dutta P. Landscape of molecular events in pituitary apoplexy. Frontiers in Endocrinology. Mar 20 2018;**9**:107

[28] Cornelius A, Cortet-Rudelli C, Assaker R, Kerdraon O, Gevaert M-H, Prévot V, et al. Endothelial expression of endocan is strongly associated with tumor progression in pituitary adenoma. Brain Pathology. 2012;**22**(6):757-764

[29] Tanase C, Popescu ID, Mihai S, Necula L, Cruceru ML, Hinescu ME. Decreased expression of APAF-1 and increased expression of cathepsin B in invasive pituitary adenoma. Oncotargets and Therapy. Dec 22 2014;**8**:81-90

[30] Yang Q, Li X. Molecular network basis of invasive pituitary adenoma: A

review. Frontiers in Endocrinology. Jan 24 2019;**10**:7

[31] Wang X, Fang Y, Zhou Y, Guo X, Ke X, Li C, et al. SDF-1α/MicroRNA-134 axis regulates nonfunctioning pituitary neuroendocrine tumor growth via targeting VEGFA. Frontiers in Endocrinology. Dec 9 2020;**11**. DOI 10.3389/fendo.2020.566761

[32] Xing B, Kong YG, Yao Y, Lian W, Wang RZ, Ren ZY. Study on the expression levels of CXCR4, CXCL12, CD44, and CD147 and their potential correlation with invasive behaviors of pituitary adenomas. Biomedical and Environmental Sciences. Jul 2013;**26**(7):592-598

[33] Li S, Li S, Zhang Z, Xue J, Guo X, Liang S, et al. Effect of hypoxia on DDR1 expression in pituitary adenomas. Medical Science Monitor. Aug 19 2015;**21**:2433-2438

Section 2

Modulators of Tumor Angiogenesis

Chapter 3

Role of Exosomes in Tumor Induced Neo-Angiogenesis

Joni Yadav, Nikita Aggarwal, Apoorva Chaudhary, Tanya Tripathi, Dikkshita Baruah, Suhail Chhakara, Divya Janjua, Arun Chhokar, Kulbhushan Thakur, Anna Senrung and Alok Chandra Bharti

Abstract

Exosomes are the nanovesicles, belonging to the type of extracellular vesicles (EVs), produced by normal as well as tumor cells and function as a mode in cell-to-cell communication. Tumor cells utilize various approach to communicate with neighboring cells for facilitating tumor invasion and progression, one of these approaches has been shown through the release of exosomes. Tumor-derived exosomes (TEX) have the ability to reprogram/modulate the activity of target cells due to their genetic and molecular cargo. Such exosomes target endothelial cells (among others) in the tumor microenvironment (TME) to promote angiogenesis which is an important element for solid tumor growth and metastasis. So, exosomes play a vital role in cancer invasiveness and progression by harboring various cargoes that could accelerate angiogenesis. Here first, we will present an overview of exosomes, their biology, and their role in different cancer models. Then, we will emphasis on exosomes derived from tumor cells as tumor angiogenesis mediators with a particular importance on the underlying mechanisms in various cancer origins. In the end, we will unveil the therapeutic potential of tumor derived exosomes as drug delivery vehicles against angiogenesis.

Keywords: extracellular vesicles, angiogenesis, exosomes, tumor, endothelial cells (ECs)

1. Introduction

Tumor microenvironment interacts with tumor cells, creating an environment to suppress or contribute towards tumor development and progression [1]. For the tumor development, inflammation and angiogenesis are the processes which play vital roles from initial to the advanced stages of cancer [2]. Extreme angiogenesis and neo-angiogenesis play a fundamental role in tumor progression, which is driven by various pro-and anti-angiogenic factors [3]. There are different ways for tumor cells to communicate with adjacent cells/tissues for facilitating tumor progression; one of these is through exosomes [4, 5]. Exosomes can transport various biomolecules like DNA fragments, mRNAs, noncoding RNAs, proteins, and lipids from a source cell to target/recipient cells that can enhance angiogenesis, which play a significant role in cancer progression [6]. There are evidences that various noncoding RNAs, particularly microRNAs and long non-coding RNAs (lncRNAs) play significant role in the regulation of angiogenesis [7]. Thus, alteration of angiogenesis has become a striking approach for development of effective cancer therapy [1].

2. Extracellular vesicles (EVs)

Prior to the discovery of exosomes it was assumed that the transmission of information between mammalian cells occurs in an indirect manner. In 1983, two pioneer studies carried out on the differentiation of reticulocytes into mature erythrocytes, reported release of transferrin receptors into extracellular space in form of small vesicles, which were later termed as "exosomes" by R.M. Johnstone [6, 8–10]. EVs are vesicles enclosed with phospholipid bilayer secreted in the extracellular matrix. Initially, they were initially considered as "garbage dumpsters" but now they are popularly being referred as "signal boxes" [11]. The presence of extracellular vesicles in solid tissue, physiological fluid, and cell culture supernatants has been demonstrated by a number of studies [12]. EV's are broadly categorized into different subtypes like microsomes, microvesicles, retrovirus-like particles and apoptotic bodies, different from each other on the basis of size, surface markers and their mode of biogenesis [13]. Extracellular vesicle is a collective term for exosomes and microvesicles. Microvesicles originate from through outward budding and fusion of plasma membrane whereas, exosomes are released via endocytosis and fusion with plasma membrane [14]. Exosomes are the smallest (30–100 nm) subpopulation of EVs. CD9, CD63 and Alix are the specific surface markers for these exosomes [13]. Exosome serve as important cell communication regulators and have gained more attention among all the diverse types of extracellular vesicles because they represent a more homogenous set of vesicular population more closely representing the parent cell of origin [15].

2.1 Exosome biogenesis

Exosomes are endosome derived extracellular vesicles. Multivesicular endosomes (MVEs) or multivesicular bodies (MVBs) are secreted via intracellular secretion pathway, from the plasma membrane. Early endosomes develop into MVBs which fuse with the cell membrane and release the exosomes or else undergoes degradation in lysosomes and autophagosomes. They are cup-or disc-shaped when observed under electron microscopy having a diameter of 30–150 nm [11, 16]. Various proteins and molecules like (ALIX, VPS4, and TSG101) are some of the major proteins involved in exosome biogenesis, content assembly and their secretion via endosomal sorting complex [16]. Exosome biogenesis supposedly occurs via two major pathways: Endosomal sorting complexes required for transport (ESCRT) dependent and ESCRT independent. The ESCRT dependent process includes ESCRT complex (0, I, and II) which are involved in recognizing and sequestering the ubiquitinylated proteins on the endosomal membrane. Exosomes are formed by membrane remodeling, involving bud formation by invagination of this endosomal membrane [17]. ESCRT independent pathway involves tetraspanins such as CD63 and lipid metabolism enzymes like neutral sphingomyelinase (nSMase) and rab family protein consisting of more than 60 GTPases that regulate intracellular trafficking of exosomes [16]. Anchoring of MVBs

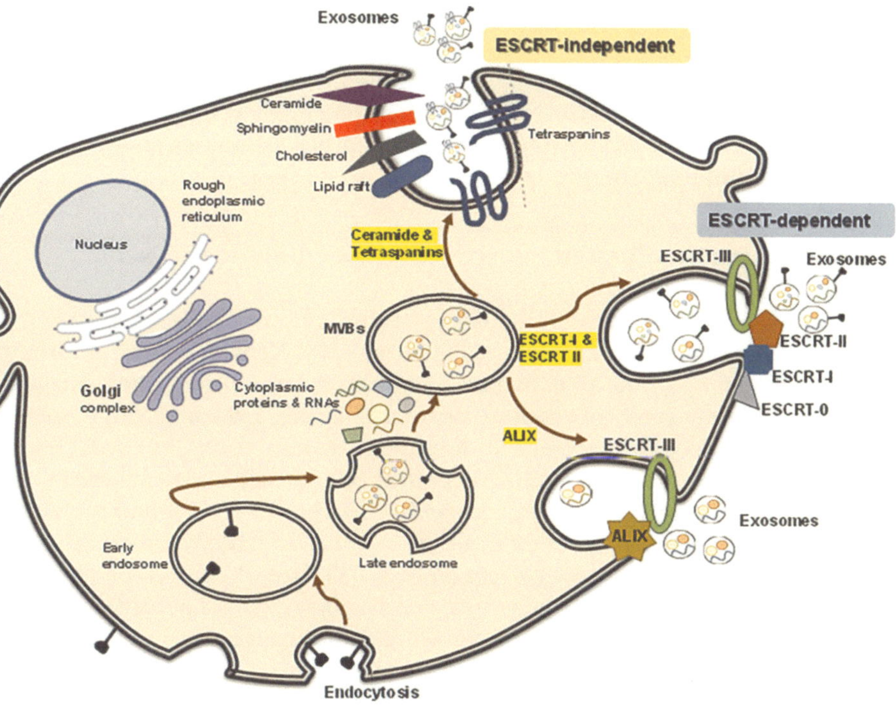

Figure 1.
Schematic representation of exosome biogenesis and secretion from eukaryotic cells. Exosome's formation starts with endocytosis, which involves inward budding of plasma membrane, leading to the formation of early and late endosomes. Further, small vesicles are generated by inward budding of late endosomes and forming multivesicular bodies (MVBs). The ultimate fate of MVBs can be either fusion with lysosome for degradation or fusion with plasma membrane to release exosomes. The exosome formation from MVBs proceeds through ESCRT-dependent and ESCRT-independent pathways. ESCRT-dependent pathway involves various ESCRT proteins like (ESCRT 0, I, II, and III) and ESCRT-independent includes lipids (ceramide) and the tetraspanins.

and transportation of different exosomes is carried out by different RAB subtypes proteins. Early endosome transportation involves RAB5 and RAB21 proteins to mediate endocytosis pathway from early to late endosome and then to lysosome for degradation involves RAB7 protein. Tumor-associated vesicle trafficking requires a vital protein that is RAB27 and it is highly expressed in several tumors. Other than this, various RAB proteins which include RAB 3,11,26,27, 35, 37 and RAB 38 are linked with the exocytic pathway of vesicle trafficking [11]. RAB27 helps in the release of exosomes from mature endosomes enriched in TSG101, ALIX and CD63 whereas RAB11 & RAB35 are associated with the release of early nuclear endosomes which are enriched with PLP, Wnt and TfR. Finally, MVBs fused with the plasma membrane and exosomes are excreted out in the extracellular environment [12]. Diagrammatic representation of exosome biogenesis and secretion has been shown in **Figure 1**.

2.2 Exosomal content

Exosomes are nanovesicles enriched with a repertoire of biomolecules like proteins, nucleic acids and lipids [16]. Exosomes are dynamic and heterogeneous in nature with respect to their content which majorly depends on their cellular origin, pathological and physiological state of the parent cells. Exosomes from different cell types are enriched specifically in proteins like Alix, Tsg101, integrins, Rab GTPases, tetraspanins (CD9) and (CD63), MHC class II proteins and heat shock proteins (HSP90, HSP70), which alsoserve as exosome marker proteins [16, 18]. Besides these, exosomes are also enriched with double-stranded DNA's and RNA population of different classes such as microRNA (miRNA), long noncoding RNA (lncRNA) [19]. ExoCarta and Vesiclepedia (http://microvesicle.org/), databases have cataloged the RNA, protein and lipid content of exosomes derived from different sources.

3. Mechanisms involved in exosomes-induced angiogenesis

Tumor derived exosomes (TEXs) have been shown to play a significant role in tumor progression by accelerating angiogenesis [20]. New blood vessel formation occurred when angiogenic signaling pathways are activated by tumor-derived exosomes, when they are up taken by normal ECs [21]. Exosomal cargo once internalized into recipient cells present in the tumor microenvironment, can regulate their fate, function, and phenotype [22, 23]. Tumor cell derived exosomal cargo can activate/inhibit the various signaling pathway in ECs via receptor-ligand interaction [24]. There are several studies represent multiple avenues in which cancer-derived exosomes exert pro-angiogenic effects on ECs. Till date, the different signaling pathways that are involved in exosomes-induced angiogenesis are poorly known. However, the exosomal cargo which is involved in tumor progression and angiogenesis have been documented. Role of TEXs cargoes which is involved in tumor angiogenesis is showed in **Figure 2**. Also, a list of all mRNAs, proteins, and noncoding RNAs which are found in TEXs for regulating tumor angiogenesis are listed in **Table 1**.

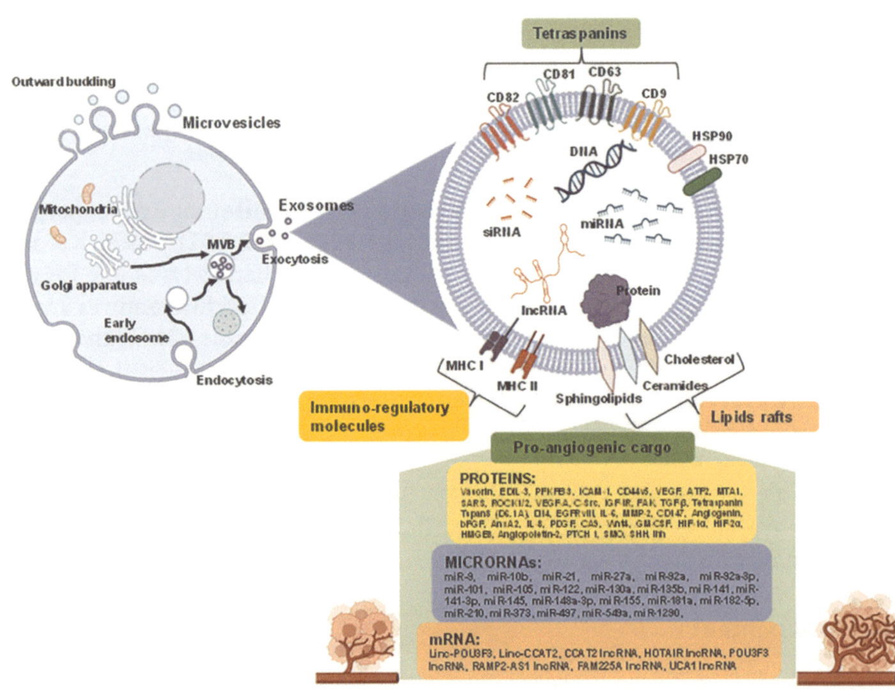

Figure 2.
Tumor derived exosomes as carrier of pro-angiogenic cargo from different cancer models promote neo-angiogenesis. Tumor-derived exosomes are enriched in proangiogenic proteins, mRNAs, miRNAs, and long noncoding RNAs which are transferred to recipient endothelial cells and activate various angiogenic signaling pathways involved in different angiogenesis process via cell proliferation, migration, and invasion.

DOI: http://dx.doi.org/10.5772/intechopen.104400

Exosomal cargo	Tumor type	Type of study (*in-vitro/ in-vivo*)	Cell lines	Target cell	Mechanisms	Function	References
EGFRVIII	Glioma cells	Both	U373Viii	U373 and HUVECs	Increase in the VEGF gene expression, by activating the MAPK and Akt pathways	Pro-angiogenesis	[25, 26]
Dll4	Glioma cells	Both	U87MG	HUVEC	Inhibition of notch signaling	Pro-angiogenesis	[27]
POU3F3 lncRNA	Glioma cells	*In-vitro*	A172, U87-MG, U251 and T98G	HBMVECs	Increasing the expression of bFGF, VEGFA and bFGFR in ECs	Pro-angiogenesis	[22]
HOTAIR lncRNA	Glioma cells	*In-vitro*	A172	HBMVECs	Increase in the VEGFA expression of ECs	Pro-angiogenesis	[28]
CCAT2 lncRNA	Glioma cells	*In-vitro*	A172, U87-MG, U251, and T98G	HUVECs	Increase in the expression of VEGFA and other angiogenic signaling molecules of ECs and decrease in the apoptosis process	Pro-angiogenesis	[29]
IL-8, PDGF	Glioblastoma	*In-vitro and ex-vivo*	U87MG	ECs	PI3K/AKT signaling	Pro-angiogenesis	[30]
VEGF-A	Glioblastoma	*In-vitro*	GSC	Brain microvascular ECs	Enhancement in angiogenic potential of brain ECs	Pro-angiogenesis	[31]
miR-148a-3p	Glioblastoma	*In-vitro*	U-138-MG, U251-MG, and HEK-293 T	HUVECs	Activating the EGFR/MAPK signaling pathway by inhibiting ERRFI1	Pro-angiogenesis	[32]
miR-182-5p	Glioblastoma	*In-vitro*	U-251MG, H4, A-172, U-118MG, LN-18, and U-87MG	HUVECs	Targeting Kruppel-like Factor 2 and 4	Pro-angiogenesis	[33]
miR-10b	Breast cancer	*In-vitro*	MCF-7 and MM-231	HMLE	Suppression of HOXD10 and KLF4 proteins level	Promotes cell invasion	[34]
miR-373	Breast cancer	*In-vitro*	MCF-7 and MM-231	ECs	Wnt/β-catenin signaling	Pro-tumorigenesis	[35]
miR-122	Breast cancer	Both	MCF-10A and MM-231	Normal cells in pre metastasic niche	Downregulation of PKM	Promotes metastasis, before angiogenesis	[36]
miR-497	Breast cancer	Both	MCF-7	HUVECs	Decrease in the expression of VEGF and HIF-1	Anti-angiogenesis	[37]
AnxA2	Breast cancer	Both	MCF10A and MM-231	Macrophages and ECs	Generation of plasmin	Pro-angiogenesis	[38]
miR-210	Breast cancer	Both	4 T1	ECs	Upregulation of VEGF	Pro-angiogenesis	[39]
miR-145	Breast cancer	Both	MDA-MB-231	HUVECs	STIM1 promotes angiogenesis by reducing exosomal miR-145 which targets IRS1	Pro-angiogenesis	[40]
NA	Breast cancer	*In-vitro*	MCF-7 and MM-231	ADSCs	SMAD pathway	Pro-angiogenesis	[41]
miR-135b	Multiple myeloma	Both	RPMI8226, KMS-11 and U266	ECs	Suppression of FIH-1	Pro-angiogenesis	[42]

Exosomal cargo	Tumor type	Type of study (*in-vitro/ in-vivo*)	Cell lines	Target cell	Mechanisms	Function	References
Angiogenin, bFGF, VEGF	Multiple myeloma	Both	ST33MMVT and RPMI8226	ECs, bone marrow stromal cells	Activation of P53, N-terminal kinase, C-jun and STAT3,	Pro-angiogenesis	[43]
miR-9	Melanoma	*Both*	SK23	ECs	JAK-STAT pathway	Pro-angiogenesis	[44]
IL-6, VEGF, and MMP-2	Melanoma	*In-vitro*	HTB63, Mewo, and A375	ECs	WNT5A signaling pathway	Pro-angiogenesis	[45]
GM-CSF, HIF-1α, HIF-2α	Melanoma	*Ex-vivo*	NA	ECs and M1/M2 macrophages	Upregulation of VEGF expression	Pro-angiogenesis	[46]
Tetraspanin Tspan8 (D6.1A)	Pancreatic cancer	Both	BSp73AS	ECs	Upregulation in the expression of MMP, VEGF, and VEGFR	Pro-angiogenesis	[47, 48]
Wnt4	Colorectal cancer	Both	HT29 and HCT116	ECs	Wnt/β-catenin pathway	Pro-angiogenesis	[49]
lncRNA UCA1	Pancreatic cancer	*In-vitro*	PANC-1, MIA PaCa-2, BxPC-3, Aspc-1, Sw1990, and HEK293T	HUVECs	AMOTL2/ERK1/2 Signaling Pathway	Pro-angiogenesis	[50]
M-phase-related transcripts	Colorectal cancer	*In-vitro*	SW480	ECs	Modulation of M-phase of cell cycle and activation of cell proliferation	Initiate angiogenesis	[51]
miR-21	Lung cancer	*In-vitro*	SV40	HUVECs	Upregulation of VEGF	Pro-angiogenesis	[52]
miR-23a	Lung cancer	*In-vitro*	NCI-H1437, H1648, H1792 and H2087	HUVECs	Exosomal miR-23a increased angiogenesis and vascular permeability by targeting prolyl hydroxylase and tight junction protein ZO-1	Pro-angiogenesis	[53]
miR-141	Small cell lung cancer	*In-vitro*	H446 and H1048	HUVECs	Exosomal miR-141/KLF12 pathway	Pro-angiogenesis	[54]
Profilin 2	Small cell lung cancer	*In-vitro*	H446	HUVECs	t PFN2 activated Smad2/3 in H446 and pERK in ECs	Pro-angiogenesis	[55]
Vasorin	Hepatocellular carcinoma	*In vitro*	HepG2	HUVEC	Promote cell proliferation and migration	Pro-angiogenesis	[56]
Angiopoietin-2	Hepatocellular carcinoma	Both	Hep3B, SNU182, SNU387, Li7 and MHCC97H	HUVECs	Tie2-independent pathway	Pro-angiogenesis	[57]
miR-1290	Hepatocellular Carcinoma	*In-vitro*	Hep3 B and HepG2	HUVECs	miR-1290-Induced proangiogenic phenotype via targeting SMEK1	Pro-angiogenesis	[58]
NA	Renal cancer	*In-vitro*	786-0	HUVEC	Upregulation of VEGF, expression and downregulation of hepaCAM	Pro-angiogenesis	[59]
NA	Renal cancer	*In-vitro*	786-0	786-0	Increase in the expression of CXCR4 and MMP-9	Enhance migration and invasion	[60]
CA9	Renal cancer	*In-vitro*	786-0	HUVEC	Increasing the MMP-2 expression	Pro-angiogenesis	[61]

Exosomal cargo	Tumor type	Type of study (*in-vitro/ in-vivo*)	Cell lines	Target cell	Mechanisms	Function	References
miR-549a	Renal cancer	Both	786-0 and 293T	HUVECs	Exosomal miR-549a affects angiogenesis and endothelial cell migration by silencing HIF1α in HUVECs	Pro-angiogenesis	[62]
miR-27a	Renal clear cell carcinoma	*In-vitro*	786-0, RPTEC and HEK293T	HUVECs	RCCC-derived miR-27a-loaded exosomes inhibit SFRP1 expression and accelerate tumor angiogenesis in RCCC	Pro-angiogenesis	[63]
EDIL-3	Bladder cancer	*In-vitro*	TCC-SUP, T24, and SV-HUC	HUVEC	Promote cell proliferation and migration	Pro-angiogenesis	[24]
miR-181a	Papillary thyroid cancer (PTC)	Both	BCPAP and K1	HUVECs	Hypoxic PTC-secreted exosomes delivered miR-181a that inhibits DACT2 via downregulating MLL3, leading to YAP-VEGF-mediated angiogenesis	Pro-angiogenesis	[64]
miR-21	Head and neck squamous cell carcinoma	Both	FaDu	$CD14^{+}$ human monocytes	Increasing the expression of M2 polarization markers of TAMs	Pro-angiogenesis	[65]
ICAM-1, CD44v5	Nasopharyngeal carcinoma	*In-vitro*	C666-1, NP69 and NP460	HUVEC	Src kinase, ERK1/2 kinase, p38 MAPK, RhoA/ROCK, and eNOS	Pro-angiogenesis	[66]
PFKFB-3	Nasopharyngeal carcinoma	*In-vitro*	CNE2	HUVEC	Increasing in the production of Fru-2,6-P2 and lactate	Pro-angiogenesis	[67]
HMGB3	Nasopharyngeal carcinoma	Both	CNE1, CNE2, 5-8 F, 6-10B and NP69	HUVECs	HMGB3-containing nEXOs accelerated angiogenesis in vitro and in vivo	Pro-angiogenesis	[68]
FAM225A lncRNA	Esophageal squamous cell carcinoma cells	*In-vitro*	ECA109, TE-1, KYSE150, and KYSE-410, and HET-1A	HUVECs	Sponging miR-206 thus derepressing its targets NETO2 and FOXP1 thereby activating PI3K/Akt/NF-κB/Snail axis	Pro-angiogenesis	[69]
miR-130a	Gastric cancer	Both	SGC-7901	HUVEC	Downregulation of c-MYB	Pro-angiogenesis	[70]
NA	Chronic myeloid leukemia	Both	K562	HUVEC	Src pathway	Pro-angiogenesis	[71]
IL-8	Chronic myeloid leukemia	Both	LAMA84	HUVEC	MAPK signaling	Pro-angiogenesis	[72]
miR-92a	Chronic myeloid leukemia	*In-vitro*	K562	ECs	Targeting integrin-α5	Pro-angiogenesis	[73]
miR-210	Chronic myeloid leukemia	*In-vitro*	K562	ECs	Downregulation of EFNA3	Pro-angiogenesis	[74]
miR-21	Chronic myeloid leukemia	Both	K562 LAMA84	HUVEC	Downregulation of RhoB	Anti-angiogenesis	[75]
TGF-β	Prostate cancer	*In-vitro*	LNCAP, DU145, and PC3	Fibroblasts	SMAD-dependent signaling	Pro-angiogenesis and pro-tumorigenesis	[76]

Exosomal cargo	Tumor type	Type of study (*in-vitro*/ *in-vivo*)	Cell lines	Target cell	Mechanisms	Function	References
C-Src, IGF-IR, FAK	Prostate cancer	*In-vitro*	DU145, PC3 and C4-2B	ECs	Upregulation of VEGF	Pro-angiogenesis	[77]
VEGF	Ovarian cancer	*In-vitro*	CABAI	HUVEC	Acts through its tyrosine kinase receptors	Pro-angiogenesis	[78]
CD147	Ovarian cancer	*In-vitro*	CABAI, A2780, OVCAR3 and SKOV3	HUVEC	Upregulation of MMP and VEGF	Pro-angiogenesis	[79]
ATF2, MTA1, SARS, ROCK1/2	Ovarian cancer	*In-vitro*	CAOV3	HUVEC	Upregulation of VEGF and HIF-1α	Pro-angiogenesis	[80]
miR-221-3p	Cervical cancer	*In-vitro*	CasKi, SiHa, HeLa and SW756	MVECs	CC cells-derived exosomes harboring miR-221-3p enhanced MVEC angiogenesis in CC by decreasing MAPK10	Pro-angiogenesis	[81]
miR-141-3p	Ovarian cancer	*In-vitro*	SKOV-3a	HUVECs	Activating the JAK/STAT3 and NF-κB signaling pathways	Pro-angiogenesis	[82]
PTCH 1, SMO, SHH, Ihh	Cervical cancer	*In-vitro*	SiHa, HeLa and C33a	HUVECs	CC cells-derived exosomes promote pro-angiogenic response in endothelial cells via upregulation of Hh-GLI signaling and modulate downstream angiogenesis-related target genes	Pro-angiogenesis	[83, 84]
TIE2	Cervical cancer	*In-vitro*	SiHa, HeLa and THP1	HUVECs	TIE2-high tumor cells deliver TIE2 to macrophages to induce TIE2-expressing macrophages via exosomes	Pro-angiogenesis	[85]
RAMP2-AS1 lncRNA	Chondrosarcoma cells	*In-vitro*	SW1353	HUVECs	Sponging miR-2355-5p thus derepressing its target VEGFR2 thereby increasing angiogenic cell surface receptors	Pro-angiogenesis	[86]
miR-92a-3p	Retinoblastoma	Both	WERI-Rb1	HUVECs	Exosomally delivered miR-92a-3p modulates angiogenesis by targeting KLF2	Pro-angiogenesis	[87]
miR-155	Burkitt's lymphoma	*In-vitro*	Raji	ARPE-19	Upregulation of VEGF-A expression via VHL/HIF-1α pathway	Pro-angiogenesis	[88]

Abbreviations: *AnxA2: annexin A2; ATF2: alcohol acetyltransferase II; BMSCs: bone marrow stromal cells; bFGF: basic fibroblast growth factor; bFGFR: basic fibroblast growth factor receptor; CXCR4: C-X-C chemokine receptor type 4; CA9: carbonic anhydrase 9; DLL4: delta-like 4; ECs: endothelial cells; EVs: extracellular vesicles; ESCRT: endosomal sorting complex for transport; EGFR/MAPK: epidermal growth factor receptor/mitogen-activated protein kinase; ERRFI1: ERBB receptor feedback inhibitor 1; eNOS: endothelial nitric oxide synthase; EFNA3: ephrin-A3; EGFRVIII: epidermal growth factor receptor VIII; FIH-1: factor inhibiting HIF-1; FOXP1: forkhead box protein P1; FAK: focal adhesion kinase; GM-CSF: granulocyte-macrophage colony stimulating factor; HUVECs: human umbilical vein endothelial cells; HBMVECs: human brain microvascular endothelial cells; HCC: hepatocellular carcinoma; HNC: head and neck cancer; HIF-1: hypoxia-inducible factor-1; HOXD10: homeobox Protein Hox-D10; HIF1α: hypoxia-inducible factor-1α; HMGB3: high mobility group protein B3; IRS1: insulin receptor substrate 1; IL-8: interleukin 8; ICAM-1: intercellular adhesion molecule 1; IGF-IR: insulin-like growth factor-I receptor; Ihh: Indian hedgehog homolog; JAK-STAT: Janus tyrosine kinase-signal transducer and activator of transcription; KLF4: Krueppel-like factor 4; KLF12: Krueppel-like factor 12; lncRNAs: long non-coding RNAs; MVEs: multivesicular endosomes; MVBs: multivesicular bodies; MAPK: mitogen-activated protein kinase; MMP: matrix metalloproteinase; MTA1: metastasis-associated protein 1; NPC: nasopharyngeal carcinoma; nEXOs: nuclear exosomes; PTC: papillary thyroid cancer; PUFA: polyunsaturated omega-3 fatty acid; PI3K: phosphoinositide 3-kinases; PKM: M2-pyruvate kinase; PFN2: profilin-2; PI3K/Akt/NF-κB: phosphoinositide 3-kinases/Akt/nuclear factor-κB; PDGF: platelet derived growth factor; PFKFB-3: 6-phosphofructo-2-kinase/fructose-2,6-bisphosphatase 3; PTCH 1: protein patched homolog 1; RCC: renal cell carcinoma; RCCC: renal clear cell carcinoma; RhoA/ROCK: Ras homolog family member A/Rho-associated kinase; ROCK1/2: Rho-associated kinase ½; SCLC: small cell lung cancer; siRNAs: small interfering RNAs; STIM1; stromal-interacting molecule 1; STAT3: signal transducer and activator of transcription 3; SMEK1: suppressor of MEK protein; SFRP1: secreted frizzled-related protein 1; SARS: severe acute respiratory syndrome; SMO: smoothened; SHH: sonic hedgehog; TEX: tumor-derived exosomes; TME: tumor microenvironment; tPA: tissue plasminogen activator; TGF-β: transforming growth factor β; VEGFA: vascular endothelial growth factor A; VEGFR: vascular endothelial growth factor receptor; VHL/HIF-1α: Von Hippel-Lindau/hypoxia inducible factor-1α; YAP-VEGF: yes-associated protein-vascular endothelial growth factor; ZO-1: zona occludens 1.*

Table 1.
Tumor derived exosomes as carrier of pro-angiogenic cargo from different cancer models promotes neo-angiogenesis.

3.1 Glioblastoma

Exosomes derived from glioblastoma cells are known to carry different mRNAs, miRNAs and angiogenic factors which interacts with ECs and thus stimulate angiogenesis. Kucharzewska et al. demonstrated export of pro-angiogenic factors IL-8 and PDGF through exosomes derived from the hypoxic glioma cells and thus induce endothelial proliferation and cell migration by activating the PI3K/AKT signaling pathway [30]. Exosomes from glioblastoma cells showed enrichment of different non-coding RNAs that include, microRNAs (miRNAs): miR-148a-3p, miR-182-5p; long non-coding RNAs (lncRNAs): POU3F3, HOTAIR, CCAT2 in the regulation of glioma cell angiogenesis [22, 28, 29, 32, 33]. Exosomes derived from glioma cells are also known to carry pro-angiogenic proteins such as EGFRvIII, VEGF-A and DII4 which are important for tumor growth, survival and angiogenesis through the activation of Akt and MAPK signaling pathways [25–27, 31].

3.2 Breast cancer

Breast cancer derived-exosomes transfer majorly pro-angiogenic microRNAs: miR-10b, miR-101, miR-105, miR-122, miR-145, miR-210 and miR-373 responsible for tumor invasion, metastasis and lead to angiogenesis [34–36, 39–41]. However, Wu et al. found that exosomes secreted from breast cancer cells loaded with miR-497 are responsible for anti-angiogenesis by downregulating the VEGF and HIF-1 [37]. Maji et al. have observed that Annexin A2 was transferred via breast cancer exosomes to ECs and induces the process of vascularization and angiogenesis through the tissue plasminogen activator (tPA)-dependent manner *in-vitro* and *in-vivo* [38].

3.3 Multiple-myeloma

Multiple myeloid cancer cells derived exosomes are known to carry miR-135b and responsible for tube formation in ECs by suppressing its target FIH-1 [42]. Wang et al. observed that various pro-angiogenic factors are released into the exosomes derived from multiple myeloma cells such as angiogenin, bFGF and VEGF that promote tumor growth [43].

3.4 Melanoma

In a study conducted by Zhuang et al. demonstrated that exogenous miR-9 can advance tumor angiogenesis by downregulating the SOCS-5 levels, which can discordantly regulate the JAK-STAT signaling pathway [44]. Hood et al. have observed exosomes released from melanoma cells stimulate the expression of HIF-1α, HIF-2α and GM-CSF, which leads to angiogenesis in endothelial cells [46]. Moreover, Ekstrom et al. showed that the WNT5A signaling promotes the exosomal secretion from melanoma cells containing immunomodulatory and pro-angiogenic factors such as IL-6, MMP-2 and VEGF [45].

3.5 Pancreatic cancer

Pancreatic adenocarcinoma produced exosomes having high levels of tetraspanin Tspan8 (D6.1A) that promote migration, proliferation and sprouting in ECs. Moreover, these exosomes also help in maturation of endothelial progenitor cells [47, 48].

Guo et al. showed that lncRNA UCA1 was exported through exosomes derived from the hypoxic pancreatic cancer cells are responsible for angiogenesis via miR-96-5p/AMOTL2 signaling pathway [50].

3.6 Colorectal cancer

Studying the exosomes from the colorectal carcinoma demonstrated that these exosomes carry pro-angiogenic factors Wnt 4, which helps in angiogenesis of ECs through Wnt/β-catenin pathway [49]. Hong et al. found that the exosomes released from SW480 colorectal cancer cell lines are loaded with M-phase related transcripts such as RAD21, CDK8, and ERH and regulate M-phase of the cell cycle and promotes proliferation and in turn enhance angiogenesis [51].

3.7 Lung cancer

Exosomes derived from small cell lung cancer (SCLC) cells are found to be enriched with miR-21 and miR-23a, which is correlated with the pro-angiogenic activities in ECs [52, 53]. A study of Mao et al. demonstrated that exosomes from SCLC cells are responsible for pro-angiogenic effect via miR-141/KLF12 pathway in targeted ECs [54]. In another recent study, Profilin2 protein was transferred from the lung cancer cells via exosomes and leads to angiogenesis by activating the t-PFN2 dependent pERK pathway in endothelial cells [55].

3.8 Hepatocellular carcinoma (HCC)

Vasorin (VASN), a type I transmembrane protein has an effective role in tumor progression and angiogenesis, was secreted by exosomes of hepatocellular carcinoma cells (HCC) and promotes the migration of HUVEC cells [56]. In another study of Xie et al. showed that angiopoietin-2 protein is transferred to ECs from HCC cells via exosomes and responsible for pro-angiogenesis [57]. Recently, it was found that miR-1290 is also released from the HCC cells through exosomes and responsible for angiogenesis by inducing the miR-1290 induced pro-angiogenic phenotype in endothelial cells, by targeting the SMEK1 [58].

3.9 Renal cell carcinoma (RCC)

Zhang et al. demonstrated that exosomes derived from renal cancer cell enhances angiogenesis by upregulating the expression of VEGF and downregulating the hepaCAM expression in ECs [59]. Moreover, exosomes derived from renal cancer 786-0 cells promotes invasion and migration of the endothelial cells through upregulation of chemokine receptors CXCR4 and MMP-9 [60]. A recent study of Hou et al. observed that the exosomes derived from renal clear cell carcinoma (RCCC) are loaded with miR-27a and inhibits SFRP1 expression which leads to accelerated angiogenesis in HUVECs [63].

3.10 Bladder cancer

Beckham et al. observed that the exosomes derived from urine of patients with bladder cancer and high-grade bladder cancer cell lines contain an angiogenic factor. Epidermal growth factor (EGF)-like repeats and discoidin I-like domain-3 (EDIL-3) that facilitate cell proliferation and migration which leads to angiogenesis in endothelial cells. EDIL-3 activated EGFR signaling overrule this EDIL-3 induced bladder cell migration [24].

3.11 Papillary thyroid cancer (PTC)

In a recent study by Wang et al. observed that miR-181a is delivered by hypoxic PTC-secreted exosomes inhibits DACT2 by downregulating MLL3, leading to YAP-VEGF-mediated angiogenesis by increasing proliferation and forming capillary-like network in HUVECs. Further, angiogenic potential of hypoxic PTC-secreted exosomes was confirmed in-vivo, which was reversed in presence of hypoxic miR-181 inhibitor [64].

3.12 Head and neck cancer (HNC)

Chan et al. showed that nasopharyngeal carcinoma (NPC) derived exosomes are supplemented with pro-angiogenic factors, ICAM-1 and CD44v5, which helps in angiogenesis of endothelial cells [66]. In another study by Gu et al. recognized a vital role of PFKFB-3 in NPC derived exosomes, which helps in migration, proliferation and angiogenesis of HUVECs [67]. Exosomes derived from FaDu cells are highly enriched with miR-21, captured by monocytes present in the TME and responsible for increasing the expression of M2 polarization of TAMs markers, which helps in tumor progression by regulating the tumor invasiveness and angiogenesis [65]. In a recent study, it was observed that a nuclear protein HMGB3 is transferred to endothelial cells via exosomes released from NPC cells and responsible for accelerated angiogenesis *in-vitro* and *in-vivo* [68].

3.13 Esophageal squamous cell carcinoma (OSCC)

Zhang et al. demonstrated that exosomes released from esophageal squamous cells are enriched with lncRNA FAM225A, which accelerates esophageal squamous cell carcinoma progression and angiogenesis by sponging miR-206. Further, they showed the upregulation of NETO2 and FOXP1 expression when FAM225A absorbed the miR-206 thereby activating PI3K/Akt/NF-κB/Snail axis [69].

3.14 Gastric cancer

Exosomes derived from gastric cancer cell are enriched with miR-130a and plays a central role in tumor angiogenesis. They showed that exosomal miR-130a is able to facilitate angiogenesis by downregulating the c-MYB, which is an important transcription factor in different biological processes [70]. In another study by Li et al. demonstrated that exosomes released from irradiated gastric cancer cells promote invasiveness and proliferation of endothelial cells [89].

3.15 Chronic myeloid leukemia (CML)

LAMA84 a human CML cell line releases exosomes and are able to trigger diverse signaling pathways in ECs, leading to enhanced expression of important angiogenic factor IL-8 [72]. Umezu et al. observed that exosomes from leukemia cells can transport miR-92a into ECs and responsible for enhanced tube formation and migration by downregulation of integrin-α_5 [73]. In another study, it was found that leukemia cell derived exosomes are able to induce tube formation in HUVECs by activating Src [71]. It has been observed that exosomes released from K562 leukemia cells are loaded with miR-210 downregulate the receptor tyrosine kinase ligand, Ephrin A3 (EFNA3) [74]. However, in contrast, Taverna et al. showed that curcumin treatment deeply changes the molecular properties of exosomes released by leukemia cells, in particular, deplete the exosomes of the pro-angiogenic proteins and leads to enrichment of proteins with anti-angiogenic activity and miR-21 [75].

3.16 Prostate cancer

Exosomes derived from prostate cancer cells are known to carry TGF-β1 protein, which can induce the differentiation of recipient fibroblasts to myofibroblasts [76]. In a study by DeRita et al., showed that prostate cancer cell exosomes were loaded with, IGF-IR, FAK and c-src, which could promote tumor angiogenesis [77].

3.17 Ovarian cancer

Taraboletti et al. demonstrated that exosomes from ovarian cancer cells are known to carry pro-angiogenic growth factor VEGF, which helps in interaction between tumor and endothelial cells and is very important for angiogenesis [78]. Ovarian cancer exosomes are enriched with pro-angiogenic protein CD147, ATF 2, MTA1, SARS and ROCK1/2. They observed that these proteins can enhance the expression of vital angiogenic factors like VEGF, HIF-1α and MMPs and resulting in the enhanced angiogenesis of HUVECs [79, 80]. Additionally, Masoumi-Dehghi et al. observed that exosomes from ovarian cancer cells are enriched in miR141-3p, which helps in angiogenesis by activating the JAK/STAT and NF-kB signaling pathways [82].

3.18 Chondrosarcoma

Cheng et al. demonstrated that microarray analysis revealed that exosomes released from chondrosarcoma cells carried lncRNA RAMP2-AS1, which promotes HUVECs migration, proliferation, and tube formation which leads to angiogenesis through miR-2355-5p/VEGFR2 axis, thereby regulating the angiogenic ability of endothelial cells. Successive experiments showed that RAMP2-AS1 knockdown could decrease the pro-angiogenic effect of exosomes released from chondrosarcoma cells [86].

3.19 Retinoblastoma

Recently a study conducted by Chen et al. demonstrated that exosomes released by human retinoblastoma cell line WERI-Rb1, were enriched inmiR-92a-3p. The study, predicted that Krüppel-like factor 2 (KLF2) might activate target of miR-92a-3p, using bioinformatics tools & analysis. Thus, exosomal miR-92a-3p was found to modulate tumor angiogenesis by targeting KLF2 [87].

3.20 Burkitt's lymphoma

A study performed by Yoon et al. observed that miR-155 is transported from EBV-positive Burkitt's lymphoma cells derived exosomes which could induces angiogenesis in retinal epithelial pigment (RPE) cells (ARPE-19) by upregulation of transcriptional and translational levels of VEGF A via VHL/HIF-1α pathway. Thus, study demonstrated that miR-155 accumulation through exosomes affect nearby recipient cells [88].

3.21 Cervical cancer

Zhang et al. observed that exosomes released from cervical cancer cells harboring miR-221-3p, which accelerate the MVEC migration, proliferation, invasion and angiogenesis in cervical cancer cells by regulating MAPK10 [81]. In another study performed by Bhat et al. showed that cervical cancer exosomes were highly enriched with upstream proteins of hedgehog-GLI signaling includes, PTCH1, SMO, SHH and Ihh [83]. Also, they observed that these cervical cancer exosomes facilitate pro-angiogenic endothelial reconditioning through transfer of Hedgehog-GLI signaling components [84].

4. Therapeutic potential of tumor-exosomes in angiogenesis

The discovery of exosomes as natural carriers of different mRNAs, miRNAs and lncRNAs makes them a suitable candidate as therapeutic drug vehicles and drug carriers to target cancer cells and modulation of tumor microenvironment. Recent advance in the field reveals several success stories (**Table 2**). The manipulation of

Exosomal cargos	Study models	Study Outcome	References
let-7a miR	Breast cancer	Secreted exosomes delivered miR-let7a to the breast cancer cells expressing EGFR and inhibited cancer growth by blocking angiogenesis	[90]
HGF siRNA	Gastric cancer	Exosomes decrease the tumor growth and angiogenesis in gastric cancer by delivering hepatocyte growth factor siRNA (HGF siRNA)	[91]
Antisense RNA targeted to miR-150	NA	Downregulated the expression levels of VEGF in mice and blocked angiogenesis	[92]
miR-21, miR-23b, miR-27a/b, miR-320b, let-7 and let-7a	Breast cancer	DHA treated exosomes have altered miRNA content that have anti-angiogenic properties in breast cancer	[93]
miR-340	Old Bone Marrow Stromal Cells (BMSCs)	Exosomes having miR-340, inhibits angiogenesis through HGF/c-MET signaling pathway in ECs	[94]
miR-21	Chronic Myeloid Leukemia (CML)	Exosomes transferred miR-21 to ECs and downregulated the expression of RhoB	[75]

Abbreviations: *HGF: hepatocyte growth factor; EGFR: epidermal growth factor receptor; VEGF: vascular endothelial growth factor; DHA: docosahexaenoic acid; RhoB: Ras homolog family member B.*

Table 2.
Engineered exosomes as anti-angiogenic drug carriers in different cancer models.

exosomes as drug carriers provides significant advantage for example their nonimmunogenic nature [95]. Exosomes are also known to carry different cell surface molecules due to which they have a commendable ability to transgress numerous biological barriers, such as the BBB (blood-brain barrier). They are highly stable in blood, which permits them to perform long distance intercellular communication [96]. Clinical data from various studies revealed that progression of cancer can be delayed or prevented when tumor angiogenesis is blocked [97]. So, angiogenesis during tumor development has now become the major emphasis of study and angiogenesis inhibition is evolving as a new method to treat cancer [98]. Recent investigations reported that exosomes can decrease or increase angiogenesis based on their molecular content. Thus, there is a lot of promise in developing engineered exosomes to transport numerous biological and synthetic genetic materials that can modify the expression of various genes involved in tumor angiogenesis [99]. For example, Ohno et al. demonstrated that modified exosomes carrying EGF or GE11 on their surface can deliver miR let-7a (tumor suppressor miR) to EGFR expressing breast cancer cells in RAG2−/− mice model. Their previous investigation showed that GE11-exosomes which delivered miR-let 7a, effectively downregulated HMGA2 expression in cancer cells [90]. This study verifies that exosomes can be used as drug delivery vehicle to transport their cargo efficiently to the target cells. Exosomes have capability to act as carriers for delivering different small interfering RNAs (siRNAs) for targeted cancer treatment. Exosomes having HGF siRNA packed inside them can be transported into gastric cancer cells, where they downregulate the HGF expression [91]. Liu et al. demonstrated that exosomes are able to transport antisense RNA targeted to miR-150, which induces the expression of VEGF. They established that the neutralization of miR-150 downregulates the VEGF levels in mice and blocked angiogenesis [92]. Gupta et al. have shown that the bone marrow stromal cells (BMSCs) are involved in the tumor progression by secreting different pro-angiogenic factors, bFGF and VEGF [100]. In another study, it was observed that the miR content of exosomes derived from old and young BMSCs was different from each other. Young BMSC exosomes were highly enriched with miR-340, which inhibited the angiogenesis through HGF/c-MET signaling pathway in ECs. The antiangiogenic effect of older BMSCs was remarkably enhanced, when miR-340 was transferred to older BMSC exosomes that was highly expressed in young BMSC exosomes. Therefore, this investigation indicates the exosome-based cancer therapy via replenishment of miRNAs of exosomes [94]. The Arg-Gly-Asp (RGD) sequence containing peptide specifically bounds to αVβ3 integrin and plays an important role in endothelial cell survival, migration and angiogenic growth. In a study performed by Wang et al. showed successful binding of the RGD sequence containing peptide to the exosomal membrane surface and thereby binding of the αVβ3 integrin on the surface of angiogenic blood vessel. Thus, engineered exosomes are emerging as a new probable therapeutic motor for angiogenesis therapy [99]. In another study, it has been observed that curcumin treated CML cells released the exosomes, which are highly enriched with miR-21, which is further transferred to ECs and downregulates the expression of RhoB [75]. Docosahexaenoic acid (DHA) is a polyunsaturated omega-3 fatty acid (PUFA) and popularly known for its anti-cancer and anti-angiogenesis properties. A group of researchers demonstrated that exosomes released from the DHA-treated breast cancer cell lines are highly enriched with miRs, including miR-21, miR-27a/b, miR-23b, miR-320b, let-7 and let-7a, which are well known for their anti-angiogenic properties. They observed the increased expression of these miRs when exosomes were co-incubated with the endothelial cells. Collectively, the exosomes show a strong therapeutic potential as natural nano carrier [93].

5. Conclusion

Herein, we have emphasized the current advances in the roles of tumor derived exosomes in cancers of different origins in tumor angiogenesis. Exosomes could modulate the angiogenic programming in target cells by transferring the angiogenic cargoes that include different mRNAs, miRNAs, lncRNAs and proteins. Angiogenesis is a very complex process in which aberrant growth of tumor and its metastasis occurs. So, the inhibition of angiogenesis is a pivotal point to control the progression of cancer. In spite of increasing amount of information about tumor derived exosomal cargo and changes prompted by them on target cells, the complexity of exosomal cargoes remains to be fully elucidated. There are several limitations and road blockers in the significance of exosomes in cancer therapy. These specifically pertain to exosomal yield, exosomes efficacy and specificity of targeting for effective cancer therapy. This field is yet elusive to assess the effect of exosomes on tumor angiogenesis and use them as potential means for different cancer therapies. So, future investigations should focus on identifying the fundamental exosomal cargoes and the mechanisms behind differential loading of different bioactive molecules, whose role could be implemented for designing non-invasive procedures to detect exosomes for cancer diagnosis and prognosis as well as development of effective therapeutic approaches based on exosomes.

Acknowledgements

Not Applicable.

Funding

Financial support from Science and Engineering Research Board Department of Science and Technology, Government of India (DST-SERB (EMR/2017/004018/BBM)) and Institution of Eminence University of Delhi (Ref. No./IoE/2021/12/FRP) to ACB and grant from CCRH to ACB:SC:KT (17-51/2016–2017/CCRH/Tech/Coll./DU-Cervical Cancer.4850) and Indian Council of Medical Research (ICMR-ICRC (No.5/13/4/ACB/ICRC/2020/NCD-III), are thankfully acknowledged. Study was partly supported by Junior Research Fellowship to TT (764/(CSIR-UGC NET JUNE 2019) and Senior Research Fellowship to AC [573(CSIR-UGC NET JUNE 2017)] by University Grants Commission (UGC), Senior Research Fellowship to NA (09/045(1622)/2019-EMR-I) and JY (09/045(1629)/2019-EMR-I) by Council of Scientific and Industrial Research (CSIR); Junior Research Fellowship to DJ (09/0045/(11635)/2021-EMR-1) and AC (09/0045(12901)/2022-EMR-1).

Conflicts of interest

The authors declare that there are no competing/conflicts of interest.

Author details

Joni Yadav, Nikita Aggarwal, Apoorva Chaudhary, Tanya Tripathi, Dikkshita Baruah, Suhail Chhakara, Divya Janjua, Arun Chhokar, Kulbhushan Thakur, Anna Senrung and Alok Chandra Bharti*
Molecular Oncology Laboratory, Department of Zoology, University of Delhi (North Campus), Delhi, India

*Address all correspondence to: alokchandrab@yahoo.com

References

[1] Javan MR, Khosrojerdi A, Moazzeni SM. New insights into implementation of mesenchymal stem cells in cancer therapy: Prospects for anti-angiogenesis treatment. Frontiers in Oncology. 2019;**9**:840

[2] Aguilar-Cazares D, Chavez-Dominguez R, Carlos-Reyes A, Lopez-Camarillo C, Hernadez, de la Cruz ON, Lopez-Gonzalez JS. Contribution of angiogenesis to inflammation and cancer. Frontiers in Oncology. 2019;**9**:1399

[3] Jaszai J, Schmidt MHH. Trends and challenges in tumor anti-angiogenic therapies. Cell. 2019;**8**(9):1102. Available from: https://www.ncbi.nlm.nih.gov/pmc/articles/PMC6770676/pdf/cells-08-01102.pdf

[4] Dominiak A, Chelstowska B, Olejarz W, Nowicka G. Communication in the cancer microenvironment as a target for therapeutic interventions. Cancers (Basel). 2020;**12**(5):1232. Available from: https://www.ncbi.nlm.nih.gov/pmc/articles/PMC7281160/pdf/cancers-12-01232.pdf

[5] Stec M, Baj-Krzyworzeka M, Baran J, Weglarczyk K, Zembala M, Barbasz J, et al. Isolation and characterization of circulating micro(nano)vesicles in the plasma of colorectal cancer patients and their interactions with tumor cells. Oncology Reports. 2015;**34**(5):2768-2775

[6] Dassler-Plenker J, Kuttner V, Egeblad M. Communication in tiny packages: Exosomes as means of tumor-stroma communication. Biochimica Et Biophysica Acta. Reviews on Cancer. 1873;**2020**(2):188340

[7] Zhao Z, Sun W, Guo Z, Zhang J, Yu H, Liu B. Mechanisms of lncRNA/microRNA interactions in angiogenesis. Life Sciences. 2020;**254**:116900

[8] Harding C, Heuser J, Stahl P. Receptor-mediated endocytosis of transferrin and recycling of the transferrin receptor in rat reticulocytes. The Journal of Cell Biology. 1983;**97**(2):329-339

[9] Johnstone RM, Adam M, Hammond JR, Orr L, Turbide C. Vesicle formation during reticulocyte maturation. Association of plasma membrane activities with released vesicles (exosomes). The Journal of Biological Chemistry. 1987;**262**(19):9412-9420

[10] Pan BT, Johnstone RM. Fate of the transferrin receptor during maturation of sheep reticulocytes in vitro: Selective externalization of the receptor. Cell. 1983;**33**(3):967-978

[11] Raposo G, Stoorvogel W. Extracellular vesicles: Exosomes, microvesicles, and friends. The Journal of Cell Biology. 2013;**200**(4):373-383

[12] Xie C, Ji N, Tang Z, Li J, Chen Q. The role of extracellular vesicles from different origin in the microenvironment of head and neck cancers. Molecular Cancer. 2019;**18**(1):83

[13] Zhang Y, Yu M, Tian W. Physiological and pathological impact of exosomes of adipose tissue. Cell Proliferation. 2016;**49**(1):3-13

[14] Bebelman MP, Smit MJ, Pegtel DM, Baglio SR. Biogenesis and function of extracellular vesicles in cancer. Pharmacology & Therapeutics. 2018;**188**:1-11

[15] Guo W, Gao Y, Li N, Shao F, Wang C, Wang P, et al. Exosomes: New players in cancer (review). Oncology Reports. 2017;**38**(2):665-675

[16] Colombo M, Raposo G, Thery C. Biogenesis, secretion, and intercellular interactions of exosomes and other extracellular vesicles. Annual Review of Cell and Developmental Biology. 2014; **30**:255-289

[17] Thery C, Zitvogel L, Amigorena S. Exosomes: Composition, biogenesis and function. Nature Reviews. Immunology. 2002;**2**(8):569-579

[18] Gutierrez-Vazquez C, Villarroya-Beltri C, Mittelbrunn M, Sanchez-Madrid F. Transfer of extracellular vesicles during immune cell-cell interactions. Immunological Reviews. 2013;**251**(1):125-142

[19] Valadi H, Ekstrom K, Bossios A, Sjostrand M, Lee JJ, Lotvall JO. Exosome-mediated transfer of mRNAs and microRNAs is a novel mechanism of genetic exchange between cells. Nature Cell Biology. 2007;**9**(6):654-659

[20] Kalluri R. The biology and function of exosomes in cancer. The Journal of Clinical Investigation. 2016;**126**(4): 1208-1215

[21] Whiteside TL. Tumor-derived exosomes and their role in cancer progression. Advances in Clinical Chemistry. 2016;**74**:103-141

[22] Lang HL, Hu GW, Chen Y, Liu Y, Tu W, Lu YM, et al. Glioma cells promote angiogenesis through the release of exosomes containing long non-coding RNA POU3F3. European Review for Medical and Pharmacological Sciences. 2017;**21**(5):959-972

[23] Zhang J, Li S, Li L, Li M, Guo C, Yao J, et al. Exosome and exosomal microRNA: Trafficking, sorting, and function. Genomics, Proteomics & Bioinformatics. 2015;**13**(1):17-24

[24] Beckham CJ, Olsen J, Yin PN, Wu CH, Ting HJ, Hagen FK, et al. Bladder cancer exosomes contain EDIL-3/Del1 and facilitate cancer progression. The Journal of Urology. 2014;**192**(2): 583-592

[25] Al-Nedawi K, Meehan B, Micallef J, Lhotak V, May L, Guha A, et al. Intercellular transfer of the oncogenic receptor EGFRvIII by microvesicles derived from tumour cells. Nature Cell Biology. 2008;**10**(5):619-624

[26] Manda SV, Kataria Y, Tatireddy BR, Ramakrishnan B, Ratnam BG, Lath R, et al. Exosomes as a biomarker platform for detecting epidermal growth factor receptor-positive high-grade gliomas. Journal of Neurosurgery. 2018;**128**(4): 1091-1101

[27] Sheldon H, Heikamp E, Turley H, Dragovic R, Thomas P, Oon CE, et al. New mechanism for Notch signaling to endothelium at a distance by Delta-like 4 incorporation into exosomes. Blood. 2010;**116**(13):2385-2394

[28] Ma X, Li Z, Li T, Zhu L, Li Z, Tian N. Long non-coding RNA HOTAIR enhances angiogenesis by induction of VEGFA expression in glioma cells and transmission to endothelial cells via glioma cell derived-extracellular vesicles. American Journal of Translational Research. 2017;**9**(11):5012-5021

[29] Lang HL, Hu GW, Zhang B, Kuang W, Chen Y, Wu L, et al. Glioma cells enhance angiogenesis and inhibit endothelial cell apoptosis through the release of exosomes that contain long non-coding RNA CCAT2. Oncology Reports. 2017;**38**(2):785-798

[30] Kucharzewska P, Christianson HC, Welch JE, Svensson KJ, Fredlund E, Ringner M, et al. Exosomes reflect the hypoxic status of glioma cells and

mediate hypoxia-dependent activation of vascular cells during tumor development. Proceedings of the National Academy of Sciences of the United States of America. 2013;**110**(18): 7312-7317

[31] Treps L, Perret R, Edmond S, Ricard D, Gavard J. Glioblastoma stem-like cells secrete the pro-angiogenic VEGF-A factor in extracellular vesicles. Journal of Extracellular Vesicles. 2017; **6**(1):1359479

[32] Wang M, Zhao Y, Yu ZY, Zhang RD, Li SA, Zhang P, et al. Glioma exosomal microRNA-148a-3p promotes tumor angiogenesis through activating the EGFR/MAPK signaling pathway via inhibiting ERRFI1. Cancer Cell International. 2020;**20**:518

[33] Li J, Yuan H, Xu H, Zhao H, Xiong N. Hypoxic cancer-secreted exosomal miR-182-5p promotes glioblastoma angiogenesis by targeting Kruppel-like factor 2 and 4. Molecular Cancer Research. 2020;**18**(8): 1218-1231

[34] Singh R, Pochampally R, Watabe K, Lu Z, Mo YY. Exosome-mediated transfer of miR-10b promotes cell invasion in breast cancer. Molecular Cancer. 2014;**13**:256

[35] Eichelser C, Stuckrath I, Muller V, Milde-Langosch K, Wikman H, Pantel K, et al. Increased serum levels of circulating exosomal microRNA-373 in receptor-negative breast cancer patients. Oncotarget. 2014;**5**(20):9650-9663

[36] Fong MY, Zhou W, Liu L, Alontaga AY, Chandra M, Ashby J, et al. Breast-cancer-secreted miR-122 reprograms glucose metabolism in premetastatic niche to promote metastasis. Nature Cell Biology. 2015; **17**(2):183-194

[37] Wu Z, Cai X, Huang C, Xu J. Liu A: MiR-497 suppresses angiogenesis in breast carcinoma by targeting HIF-1alpha. Oncology Reports. 2016;**35**(3): 1696-1702

[38] Maji S, Chaudhary P, Akopova I, Nguyen PM, Hare RJ, Gryczynski I, et al. Exosomal annexin II promotes angiogenesis and breast cancer metastasis. Molecular Cancer Research. 2017;**15**(1):93-105

[39] Jung KO, Youn H, Lee CH, Kang KW, Chung JK. Visualization of exosome-mediated miR-210 transfer from hypoxic tumor cells. Oncotarget. 2017;**8**(6):9899-9910

[40] Pan S, Zhao X, Shao C, Fu B, Huang Y, Zhang N, et al. STIM1 promotes angiogenesis by reducing exosomal miR-145 in breast cancer MDA-MB-231 cells. Cell Death & Disease. 2021;**12**(1):38

[41] Cho JA, Park H, Lim EH, Lee KW. Exosomes from breast cancer cells can convert adipose tissue-derived mesenchymal stem cells into myofibroblast-like cells. International Journal of Oncology. 2012;**40**(1): 130-138

[42] Umezu T, Tadokoro H, Azuma K, Yoshizawa S, Ohyashiki K, Ohyashiki JH. Exosomal miR-135b shed from hypoxic multiple myeloma cells enhances angiogenesis by targeting factor-inhibiting HIF-1. Blood. 2014;**124**(25): 3748-3757

[43] Wang J, De Veirman K, Faict S, Frassanito MA, Ribatti D, Vacca A, et al. Multiple myeloma exosomes establish a favourable bone marrow microenvironment with enhanced angiogenesis and immunosuppression. The Journal of Pathology. 2016;**239**(2): 162-173

[44] Zhuang G, Wu X, Jiang Z, Kasman I, Yao J, Guan Y, et al. Tumour-secreted miR-9 promotes endothelial cell migration and angiogenesis by activating the JAK-STAT pathway. The EMBO Journal. 2012;**31**(17):3513-3523

[45] Ekstrom EJ, Bergenfelz C, von Bulow V, Serifler F, Carlemalm E, Jonsson G, et al. WNT5A induces release of exosomes containing pro-angiogenic and immunosuppressive factors from malignant melanoma cells. Molecular Cancer. 2014;**13**:88

[46] Hood JL. Melanoma exosome induction of endothelial cell GM-CSF in pre-metastatic lymph nodes may result in different M1 and M2 macrophage mediated angiogenic processes. Medical Hypotheses. 2016;**94**: 118-122

[47] Gesierich S, Berezovskiy I, Ryschich E, Zoller M. Systemic induction of the angiogenesis switch by the tetraspanin D6.1A/CO-029. Cancer Research. 2006;**66**(14):7083-7094

[48] Nazarenko I, Rana S, Baumann A, McAlear J, Hellwig A, Trendelenburg M, et al. Cell surface tetraspanin Tspan8 contributes to molecular pathways of exosome-induced endothelial cell activation. Cancer Research. 2010;**70**(4): 1668-1678

[49] Huang Z, Feng Y. Exosomes derived from hypoxic colorectal cancer cells promote angiogenesis through Wnt4-induced beta-catenin signaling in endothelial cells. Oncology Research. 2017;**25**(5):651-661

[50] Guo Z, Wang X, Yang Y, Chen W, Zhang K, Teng B, et al. Hypoxic tumor-derived exosomal long noncoding RNA UCA1 promotes angiogenesis via miR-96-5p/AMOTL2 in pancreatic cancer. Molecular Therapy Nucleic Acids. 2020; **22**:179-195

[51] Hong BS, Cho JH, Kim H, Choi EJ, Rho S, Kim J, et al. Colorectal cancer cell-derived microvesicles are enriched in cell cycle-related mRNAs that promote proliferation of endothelial cells. BMC Genomics. 2009;**10**:556

[52] Liu Y, Luo F, Wang B, Li H, Xu Y, Liu X, et al. STAT3-regulated exosomal miR-21 promotes angiogenesis and is involved in neoplastic processes of transformed human bronchial epithelial cells. Cancer Letters. 2016;**370**(1): 125-135

[53] Hsu YL, Hung JY, Chang WA, Lin YS, Pan YC, Tsai PH, et al. Hypoxic lung cancer-secreted exosomal miR-23a increased angiogenesis and vascular permeability by targeting prolyl hydroxylase and tight junction protein ZO-1. Oncogene. 2017;**36**(34):4929-4942

[54] Mao S, Lu Z, Zheng S, Zhang H, Zhang G, Wang F, et al. Exosomal miR-141 promotes tumor angiogenesis via KLF12 in small cell lung cancer. Journal of Experimental & Clinical Cancer Research. 2020;**39**(1):193

[55] Cao Q, Liu Y, Wu Y, Hu C, Sun L, Wang J, et al. Profilin 2 promotes growth, metastasis, and angiogenesis of small cell lung cancer through cancer-derived exosomes. Aging (Albany NY). 2020;**12**(24):25981-25999

[56] Huang A, Dong J, Li S, Wang C, Ding H, Li H, et al. Exosomal transfer of vasorin expressed in hepatocellular carcinoma cells promotes migration of human umbilical vein endothelial cells. International Journal of Biological Sciences. 2015;**11**(8):961-969

[57] Xie JY, Wei JX, Lv LH, Han QF, Yang WB, Li GL, et al. Angiopoietin-2 induces angiogenesis via exosomes in human hepatocellular carcinoma. Cell

Communication and Signaling: CCS. 2020;**18**(1):46

[58] Wang Q, Wang G, Niu L, Zhao S, Li J, Zhang Z, et al. Exosomal miR-1290 promotes angiogenesis of hepatocellular carcinoma via targeting SMEK1. Journal of Oncology. 2021;**2021**:6617700

[59] Zhang L, Wu X, Luo C, Chen X, Yang L, Tao J, et al. The 786-0 renal cancer cell-derived exosomes promote angiogenesis by downregulating the expression of hepatocyte cell adhesion molecule. Molecular Medicine Reports. 2013;**8**(1):272-276

[60] Chen G, Zhang Y, Wu X. 786-0 Renal cancer cell line-derived exosomes promote 786-0 cell migration and invasion in vitro. Oncology Letters. 2014;**7**(5):1576-1580

[61] Horie K, Kawakami K, Fujita Y, Sugaya M, Kameyama K, Mizutani K, et al. Exosomes expressing carbonic anhydrase 9 promote angiogenesis. Biochemical and Biophysical Research Communications. 2017;**492**(3):356-361

[62] Xuan Z, Chen C, Tang W, Ye S, Zheng J, Zhao Y, et al. TKI-resistant renal cancer secretes low-level exosomal miR-549a to induce vascular permeability and angiogenesis to promote tumor metastasis. Frontiers in Cell and Development Biology. 2021;**9**:689947

[63] Hou Y, Fan L, Li H. Oncogenic miR-27a delivered by exosomes binds to SFRP1 and promotes angiogenesis in renal clear cell carcinoma. Molecular Therapy Nucleic Acids. 2021;**24**:92-103

[64] Wang Y, Cen A, Yang Y, Ye H, Li J, Liu S, et al. miR-181a, delivered by hypoxic PTC-secreted exosomes, inhibits DACT2 by downregulating MLL3, leading to YAP-VEGF-mediated angiogenesis. Molecular Therapy Nucleic Acids. 2021;**24**:610-621

[65] Hsieh CH, Tai SK, Yang MH. Snail-overexpressing cancer cells promote M2-like polarization of tumor-associated macrophages by delivering miR-21-abundant exosomes. Neoplasia. 2018; **20**(8):775-788

[66] Chan YK, Zhang H, Liu P, Tsao SW, Lung ML, Mak NK, et al. Proteomic analysis of exosomes from nasopharyngeal carcinoma cell identifies intercellular transfer of angiogenic proteins. International Journal of Cancer. 2015;**137**(8):1830-1841

[67] Gu M, Li L, Zhang Z, Chen J, Zhang W, Zhang J, et al. PFKFB3 promotes proliferation, migration and angiogenesis in nasopharyngeal carcinoma. Journal of Cancer. 2017; **8**(18):3887-3896

[68] Zhang K, Liu D, Zhao J, Shi S, He X, Da P, et al. Nuclear exosome HMGB3 secreted by nasopharyngeal carcinoma cells promotes tumour metastasis by inducing angiogenesis. Cell Death & Disease. 2021;**12**(6):554

[69] Zhang C, Luo Y, Cao J, Wang X, Miao Z, Shao G. Exosomal lncRNA FAM225A accelerates esophageal squamous cell carcinoma progression and angiogenesis via sponging miR-206 to upregulate NETO2 and FOXP1 expression. Cancer Medicine. 2020; **9**(22):8600-8611

[70] Yang H, Zhang H, Ge S, Ning T, Bai M, Li J, et al. Exosome-derived miR-130a activates angiogenesis in gastric cancer by targeting C-MYB in vascular endothelial cells. Molecular Therapy. 2018;**26**(10):2466-2475

[71] Mineo M, Garfield SH, Taverna S, Flugy A, De Leo G, Alessandro R, et al. Exosomes released by K562 chronic myeloid leukemia cells promote

angiogenesis in a Src-dependent fashion. Angiogenesis. 2012;**15**(1):33-45

[72] Taverna S, Flugy A, Saieva L, Kohn EC, Santoro A, Meraviglia S, et al. Role of exosomes released by chronic myelogenous leukemia cells in angiogenesis. International Journal of Cancer. 2012;**130**(9):2033-2043

[73] Umezu T, Ohyashiki K, Kuroda M, Ohyashiki JH. Leukemia cell to endothelial cell communication via exosomal miRNAs. Oncogene. 2013; **32**(22):2747-2755

[74] Tadokoro H, Umezu T, Ohyashiki K, Hirano T, Ohyashiki JH. Exosomes derived from hypoxic leukemia cells enhance tube formation in endothelial cells. The Journal of Biological Chemistry. 2013;**288**(48):34343-34351

[75] Taverna S, Fontana S, Monteleone F, Pucci M, Saieva L, De Caro V, et al. Curcumin modulates chronic myelogenous leukemia exosomes composition and affects angiogenic phenotype via exosomal miR-21. Oncotarget. 2016;7(21):30420-30439

[76] Webber J, Steadman R, Mason MD, Tabi Z, Clayton A. Cancer exosomes trigger fibroblast to myofibroblast differentiation. Cancer Research. 2010; **70**(23):9621-9630

[77] DeRita RM, Zerlanko B, Singh A, Lu H, Iozzo RV, Benovic JL, et al. c-Src, Insulin-like growth factor i receptor, G-protein-coupled receptor kinases and focal adhesion kinase are enriched into prostate cancer cell exosomes. Journal of Cellular Biochemistry. 2017;**118**(1):66-73

[78] Taraboletti G, D'Ascenzo S, Giusti I, Marchetti D, Borsotti P, Millimaggi D, et al. Bioavailability of VEGF in tumor-shed vesicles depends on vesicle burst induced by acidic pH. Neoplasia. 2006; **8**(2):96-103

[79] Millimaggi D, Mari M, D'Ascenzo S, Carosa E, Jannini EA, Zucker S, et al. Tumor vesicle-associated CD147 modulates the angiogenic capability of endothelial cells. Neoplasia. 2007;**9**(4): 349-357

[80] Yi H, Ye J, Yang XM, Zhang LW, Zhang ZG, Chen YP. High-grade ovarian cancer secreting effective exosomes in tumor angiogenesis. International Journal of Clinical and Experimental Pathology. 2015;**8**(5):5062-5070

[81] Zhang L, Li H, Yuan M, Li M, Zhang S. Cervical cancer cells-secreted exosomal microRNA-221-3p promotes invasion, migration and angiogenesis of microvascular endothelial cells in cervical cancer by down-regulating MAPK10 expression. Cancer Management and Research. 2019;**11**: 10307-10319

[82] Masoumi-Dehghi S, Babashah S. Sadeghizadeh M: MicroRNA-141-3p-containing small extracellular vesicles derived from epithelial ovarian cancer cells promote endothelial cell angiogenesis through activating the JAK/STAT3 and NF-kappaB signaling pathways. Journal of Cell Communication and Signaling. 2020; **14**(2):233-244

[83] Bhat A, Sharma A, Bharti AC. Upstream Hedgehog signaling components are exported in exosomes of cervical cancer cell lines. Nanomedicine (London, England). 2018;**13**(17): 2127-2138

[84] Bhat A, Yadav J, Thakur K, Aggarwal N, Tripathi T, Chhokar A, et al. Exosomes from cervical cancer cells facilitate pro-angiogenic endothelial reconditioning through transfer of

Hedgehog-GLI signaling components. Cancer Cell International. 2021;**21**(1):319

[85] Du S, Qian J, Tan S, Li W, Liu P, Zhao J, et al. Tumor cell-derived exosomes deliver TIE2 protein to macrophages to promote angiogenesis in cervical cancer. Cancer Letters. 2022; **529**:168-179

[86] Cheng C, Zhang Z, Cheng F, Shao Z. Exosomal lncRNA RAMP2-AS1 derived from chondrosarcoma cells promotes angiogenesis through miR-2355-5p/VEGFR2 axis. Oncotargets and Therapy. 2020;**13**:3291-3301

[87] Chen S, Chen X, Luo Q, Liu X, Wang X, Cui Z, et al. Retinoblastoma cell-derived exosomes promote angiogenesis of human vesicle endothelial cells through microRNA-92a-3p. Cell Death & Disease. 2021;**12**(7):695

[88] Yoon C, Kim J, Park G, Kim S, Kim D, Hur DY, et al. Delivery of miR-155 to retinal pigment epithelial cells mediated by Burkitt's lymphoma exosomes. Tumour Biology. 2016;**37**(1): 313-321

[89] Li G, Lin H, Tian R, Zhao P, Huang Y, Pang X, et al. VEGFR-2 inhibitor apatinib hinders endothelial cells progression triggered by irradiated gastric cancer cells-derived exosomes. Journal of Cancer. 2018;**9**(21):4049-4057

[90] Ohno S, Takanashi M, Sudo K, Ueda S, Ishikawa A, Matsuyama N, et al. Systemically injected exosomes targeted to EGFR deliver antitumor microRNA to breast cancer cells. Molecular Therapy. 2013;**21**(1):185-191

[91] Zhang H, Wang Y, Bai M, Wang J, Zhu K, Liu R, et al. Exosomes serve as nanoparticles to suppress tumor growth and angiogenesis in gastric cancer by delivering hepatocyte growth factor siRNA. Cancer Science. 2018;**109**(3): 629-641

[92] Liu Y, Zhao L, Li D, Yin Y, Zhang CY, Li J, et al. Microvesicle-delivery miR-150 promotes tumorigenesis by up-regulating VEGF, and the neutralization of miR-150 attenuate tumor development. Protein & Cell. 2013;**4**(12):932-941

[93] Hannafon BN, Carpenter KJ, Berry WL, Janknecht R, Dooley WC, Ding WQ. Exosome-mediated microRNA signaling from breast cancer cells is altered by the anti-angiogenesis agent docosahexaenoic acid (DHA). Molecular Cancer. 2015;**14**:133

[94] Umezu T, Imanishi S, Azuma K, Kobayashi C, Yoshizawa S, Ohyashiki K, et al. Replenishing exosomes from older bone marrow stromal cells with miR-340 inhibits myeloma-related angiogenesis. Blood Advances. 2017;**1**(13):812-823

[95] Lakhal S, Wood MJ. Exosome nanotechnology: An emerging paradigm shift in drug delivery: Exploitation of exosome nanovesicles for systemic in vivo delivery of RNAi heralds new horizons for drug delivery across biological barriers. BioEssays. 2011; **33**(10):737-741

[96] Ha D, Yang N, Nadithe V. Exosomes as therapeutic drug carriers and delivery vehicles across biological membranes: Current perspectives and future challenges. Acta Pharmaceutica Sinica B. 2016;**6**(4):287-296

[97] Martinez MC, Andriantsitohaina R. Microparticles in angiogenesis: Therapeutic potential. Circulation Research. 2011;**109**(1):110-119

[98] Folkman J. Role of angiogenesis in tumor growth and metastasis. Seminars in Oncology. 2002;**29**(6 Suppl. 16):15-18

[99] Wang J, Li W, Lu Z, Zhang L, Hu Y, Li Q, et al. The use of RGD-engineered exosomes for enhanced targeting ability and synergistic therapy toward angiogenesis. Nanoscale. 2017;**9**(40): 15598-15605

[100] Gupta D, Treon SP, Shima Y, Hideshima T, Podar K, Tai YT, et al. Adherence of multiple myeloma cells to bone marrow stromal cells upregulates vascular endothelial growth factor secretion: Therapeutic applications. Leukemia. 2001;**15**(12):1950-1961

Chapter 4

Role of the IL-6/Jak/Stat Pathway in Tumor Angiogenesis: Influence of Estrogen Status

José Manuel García-Castellano, David García-Padrón, Nerea Martínez-Aragón, Margarita Ramírez-Sánchez, Vicente Vera-Gutiérrez and Leandro Fernández-Pérez

Abstract

Solid tumors, despite being hypervascularized, are hypoxic. This is due to the imbalance that exists between the inputs of the blood vessels that supply nutrients and O_2 and that remove metabolic waste products, on one side; and the demands of the tumor cells that are part of the neoplasm that is forming, on the other. From this perspective, we briefly review the sequence of morphological events that occur during neo-angiogenesis; what chemical mediators are involved in this process; and we emphasize how the IL-6/Jak/Stat signaling pathway is involved in the control of these mediators. At the same time, we review how estrogens intervene in this control procedure, and how it opens the door to understanding the mechanism of action of these mediators. This would make it possible to propose alternative treatments, which can be added to the conventional ones, and which would exploit the findings described here in the search for new antitumor therapies.

Keywords: hypoxia, solid tumor, HIF, VEG, neovascularization, Jak/Stat, estrogens

1. Introduction

Blood vessels formation is an essential activity for the proper development of the organism. The development of new blood vessels is a well-regulated process, but it is a double-edged sword. Hence, in a physiological situation, such as embryonic development, it leads to the formation of a correct vascular network directed to provide the necessary nutrients and O_2, as well as to waste products removal. However, in a tumoral scenario, is a problem since it uncontrollably feeds the tumor and provides the ways for its spread.

Paradoxically, although solid tumors are invariably hypervascularized, they contain hypoxic regions [1], with low pO_2 levels. This is because the high rate of tumor growth is greater than the rate of new vessel formation [2] and there is no balance between supply and demand. This causes neoplastic cells to be too far from a blood vessel [1], generating a nutrient and O_2 deficient state [3]. The hypoxia generated is also due to a poor O_2

diffusion and to the fact that the cells of the neo-vessels are structurally abnormal [4]. The consequence of this tumor hypoxia leads to therapeutic radio- and chemo-resistance, as well as an increased probability of generating metastatic disease [4, 5]. The cellular change towards a state of tumoral hypoxia provokes an adaptive response that facilitates cell proliferation or angiogenesis, coordinated by the activity of HIF-1α [6]. The adaptive response to hypoxia generated by HIF-1α through angiogenesis and enhanced glucose metabolism confers a survival and growth advantage to hypoxic tumor cells [7].

2. Hypoxic tumor cells generate new capillaries

Neoangiogenesis is the process by which new capillary vessels grow out of pre-existing ones (sprouting angiogenesis). These blood vessels will provide oxygen and nutrients and will remove the metabolic waste [6], which is regulated by a variety of pro- and anti-angiogenic factors [1].

The process of sprouting angiogenesis involves several sequential steps [8] that starts with the activation of endothelial cells due to diverse angiogenic stimulus, like hypoxia or inflammation [8]. The activity of endothelial cells, normally joined by adhesion molecules such as cadherins, is mediated by growth factors released after degranulation of platelet alpha granules [9, 10]. Pericytes, surrounding endothelial cells, inhibit the proliferation of the endothelial cells, also releasing cell survival signals such as VEGF and Angiopoietin-1.

As a consequence of this activation, there is a rupture of the endothelial cells tight junctions; the pericytes detach from the wall and the basement membrane, which, together with the extracellular matrix, will be degraded by activated proteases (metalloproteinases). Loss of junctions between endothelial cells allows them to invade into the surrounding interstitial tissue and, subsequently, proliferate and migrate through the matrix. These endothelial cells afterward become motile tip cells, which are located at the growing ends of the new vessels [11, 12].

Angiogenic factors, such as VEGF, increase the vascular permeability of endothelial cells, causing extravasation of plasmatic proteins and generating an extracellular matrix (ECM). In response to integrin signaling, cells migrate within that ECM, following the tip cells.

Endothelial cells move forward following the angiogenic signal sent by the tip cell that will guide them in the specific direction [12]. Adjacent cells to the tip cell will follow them, dividing to elongate the stalk and establish the lumen. This structure thus formed is an immature vessel [13].

Endothelial cells then rapidly proliferate [8], form tight and adherens junctions with other endothelial cells [11, 12], and finally, the endothelial cell migration and proliferation are inhibited.

The stabilization of the immature vessels is established by the recruitment of pericytes, which will line the capillary walls and stabilize the new vessels [11, 14]. Finally, a new extracellular matrix will be generated [15].

3. Neo-angiogenesis is a well-regulated process

The process of sprouting angiogenesis is tightly controlled by positive and negative regulators whose purpose is to control in a balanced way the structured formation of new vessels through the action of growth factors and cytokines (**Table 1**).

Factor	Function	Cell	References
HIF-1α	Transcription genes: angiogenesis; erythropoiesis; cell proliferation; energy metabolism.	Tumor cell	[16, 17]
VEGF	Stimulation of endothelial cell survival, proliferation, and motility	Tumor cells, macrophages, platelets, endothelial cells	[18]
FGF	Cell differentiation, proliferation, migration, morphogenesis, survival of endothelial cells; extracellular matrix degradation	Macrophages vascular endothelial cells	[19]
PDGF	Potent mitogen	Platelets, smooth muscle cells, activated macrophages, and endothelial cells	[20, 21]
Anp	Angiogenesis Wound healing	Pericytes, vascular endothelial cells macrophages involved in angiogenesis	[22]
HGF	HGF stimulates mitogenesis, cell motility, and matrix invasion	Endothelial cells, smooth muscles cells, bone brown-derived endothelial progenitor cells.	[23–25]
Ang	Inhibit endothelial cell proliferation and migration, tube formation, neutrophil activation and migration, monocyte and macrophage migration, leukocyte recruitment, MMP expression induces endothelial cell apoptosis and the production of anti-angiogenic factors, such as thrombospondin-1	Endothelial cells, tumor cell	[26]
Endostatin	Inhibits the migration of vascular endothelial cells Inhibiting VEGF-induced phosphorylation Apoptosis in proliferating endothelial cells	Endothelial cells	[27, 28]
PF 4	Strong angiogenesis inhibitor	Platelets	[29]
TSP-1	Inhibition of migration, proliferation, and survival of endothelial cells and the formation of capillary tubes	Platelets	[30]

Table 1.
Relationship were the most common growth factors during the neo-angiogenesis process are reported, their function, and the most common cells that produce them.

We will distinguish those factors that will improve the forming action of new vessels (enhancing factors), from those that are designed to modulate and stop the appearance or development of these vessels (inhibitory factors).

3.1 Enhancing factors

3.1.1 Hypoxia-inducible factor

Hypoxia-inducible factor (HIF-1α) is a transcription factor that regulates and coordinates the cellular response to hypoxia [31, 32], by activating genes encoding pro-angiogenic factors, such as VEGF, angiopoietin or PDGF.

When tissue and cellular oxygen levels are in a normal range, HIF-1α is degraded, disrupting the signaling cascade aimed at improving vascularization by means of pro-angiogenic factors [33].

Under low pO_2 status, HIF-1α is involved in hypoxia response by binding to canonical DNA sequences (hypoxia-responsive elements or HREs) in the promoters or enhancers of target genes [34–38]. Also, HIF-1α, through the union of hypoxia-responsive elements or HREs with the promoters of target genes, coordinates a broad response to counteract the effects of hypoxia. Under hypoxic conditions, proteasomal degradation of HIF-1α ends, and it translocates to the nucleus to activate hypoxia-inducible genes [36, 39], such as VEGF, angiopoietin, PlGF, or PDGF [40].

3.1.2 VEGF

VEGF is a glycoprotein that plays an essential role in the development of new vessels. It is produced by tumor cells, macrophages, platelets, and endothelial cells, binding to the VEGF-R1/R2 receptors present on endothelial cells. This growth factor stimulates the endothelial cells survival, proliferation, and motility, initiating the growth of new capillaries by activating the RAS/MEK/ERK pathways or the PI3K/AKT/mTOR pathway. The final effect is the stimulation of endothelial cell survival, proliferation, and motility, initiating the growth of new capillaries.

3.1.3 FGF

FGFs are a family of proteins, mostly with angiogenic effects. The best known are FGF-1 and FGF-2. They are essentially secreted by macrophages and vascular endothelial cells. They are involved in numerous processes, including the induction of endothelial cell differentiation, proliferation, migration, morphogenesis, and survival of endothelial cells; and extracellular matrix degradation by stimulating the secretion of proteases [19, 41]. FGF-1 is necessary for the differentiation and proliferation of all the cell types necessary for creating the vessel wall; while FGF-2 signaling is related to the preservation of vascular endothelial cell junctions and vessel permeability [19].

3.1.4 PDGF

Platelet-derived growth factor is a dimeric glycoprotein synthesized, stored (in the alpha granules of platelets), and released by platelets upon activation, it is also produced by other cells including smooth muscle cells, activated macrophages, and endothelial cells. PDGF is a potent mitogen for cells of mesenchymal origin.

3.1.5 Angiopoietins

Family of proteins involved in vascular repair. Ang-1 and Ang-2 are the best known. Its function is carried out by coupling an angiopoietin to its corresponding receptor (Tie-1 and Tie-2). These receptors are expressed specifically on vascular endothelial cells and on a certain type of macrophages involved in angiogenesis.

3.1.6 Hepatocyte growth factor

HGF is a factor secreted by mesenchymal cells in a paracrine manner that exerts its function through its c-Met receptor. This receptor is expressed in several cell types, such as endothelial cells, smooth muscles cells, and bone brown-derived endothelial progenitor cells. HGF stimulates mitogenesis, cell motility, and matrix invasion.

3.2 Inhibitory factors

3.2.1 Angiostatin

Angiostatin is a protein produced by autoproteolytic cleavage of certain proteins, like plasminogen. Its function is to inhibit endothelial cell proliferation and migration, tube formation, and tumor cell invasion. In addition, it decreases VEGF expression and induces endothelial cell-mediated apoptosis by thrombospondin-1.

3.2.2 Endostatin

Endostatin is a C-terminal type XVIII collagen fragment, cleaved by the proteolytic activity of MMP-7. It has anti-angiogenic activity by inhibiting FGF-2 and VEGF [1]. It also has an anti-migratory effect by binding to the α5-αv-integrins. It has the ability to directly combine to VEGFR2, inhibiting the VEGF-induced phosphorylation and consequently down-regulating receiver, as well.

3.2.3 Platelet Factor 4

It is a small protein belonging to the CXC chemokine family, usually associated with complexes with proteoglycans and released from alpha-granules of activated platelets during platelets aggregation. It is a potent inhibitor of angiogenesis, especially when acting in conjunction with the receptors of FGF2 and VEGF, leading to downstream effects on endothelial cell migration and proliferation.

3.2.4 Thrombospondin-1

TSP-1 is a glycoprotein that mediates intercellular interactions or with the ECM. This protein can bind to elements of this ECM (to fibrinogen, fibronectin, laminin, collagen types V and VII, and integrins alpha -V/beta-1), and exerts an inhibitory effect on the migration, proliferation, and survival of endothelial cells and the formation of capillary tubes.

4. Role of the IL-6/Jak/Stat pathway on the neoangiogenesis process

After a tissue injury, a cascade of events is set in motion aimed at repairing the damage. The products generated by tissue destruction stimulate the cells of the immune system. In response to this damaging process, immune cells in the tumor environment secrete multiple cytokines, such as histamine, serotonin, prostaglandins, leukotrienes; and inflammatory cytokines, such as tumor necrosis factor-α (TNF-α), interleukin-1 (IL-1), and various chemokines. Many of them belong to the IL-6 family [42]. These substances help to repair healthy tissues but nevertheless have deleterious effects on tumors.

4.1 IL-6/Jak/Stat pathway

Janus kinase (Jak), the signal activation transducer (Stat) pathway, is recognized as an evolutionarily conserved signaling pathway (**Figure 1**). After binding the

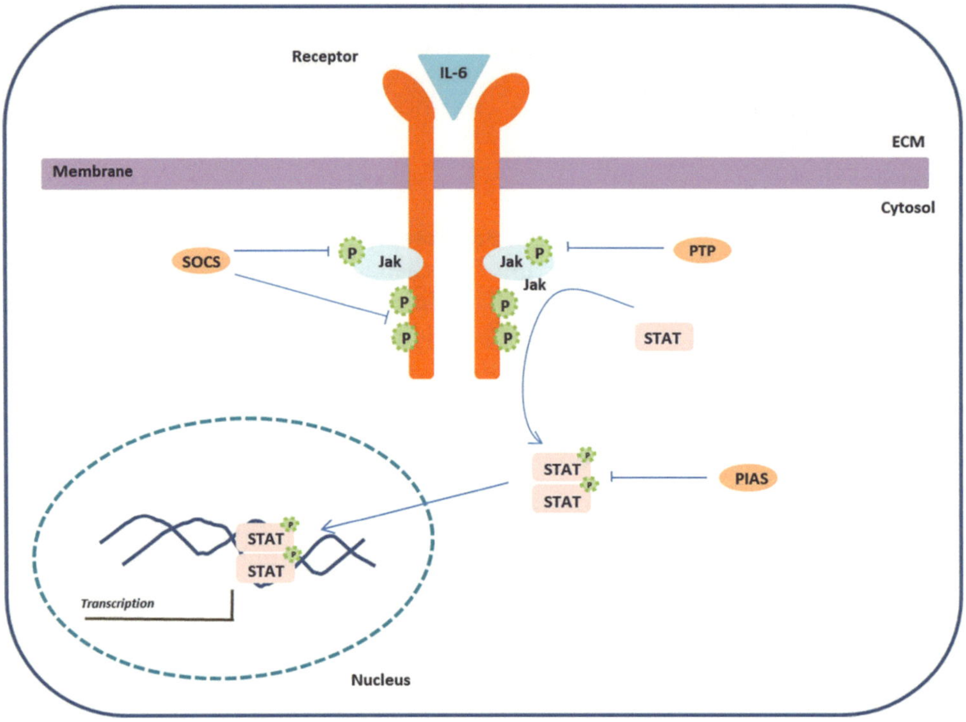

Figure 1.
IL-6/Jak/Stat pathway. After binding the cytokine to the receptor, Jak is activated by the specific tyrosine residues phosphorylation. Phosphorylated Jak, in turn, induces the phosphorylation of Stat, which, after dimerization, translocate into the nucleus where it regulates the transcription of numerous genes.

cytokine to the receptor, Jak is activated by the specific tyrosine residues phosphorylation. Phosphorylated Jak in turn induces the phosphorylation of Stat, which, after dimerization, translocate into the nucleus where it regulates the transcription of numerous genes [43].

The IL-6/Jak/Stat pathway is overexpressed in various tumors, causing continuous transcription of cell growth factors that promote tumor progression. However, this pathway not only regulates aspects such as tumor proliferation, survival, and invasion, but also contributes significantly to tumor neo-angiogenesis [44, 45], enhancing endothelial cells survival, infiltration of the ECM by immune cells followed by activation of mesenchymal cells, and finally the generation of metastases [46].

Jak/Stat is activated upon stimulation by IL-6, among several effectors, promoting endothelial cell migration and tumor angiogenesis. This function is suppressed when Jak inhibitors are administered, ending the observed endothelial cell migration *in vitro* [47].

Regulation of tumor angiogenesis is dependent on VEGF and HIF-1α transcription by endothelial cells [48–50]. This action is induced by tumor IL-6 and mediated by Stat3 [51]. These results are validated by the fact that the aberrant expression of Stat3 causes an increase in the expression level of HIF- 1α and VEGF, as well as of the metalloproteinases MMP-9 and MMP-7, enhancing tumor progression and aggressiveness [52]. This pathway is reciprocally enhanced by the action of IL-6 secreted by endothelial cells on tumor cells [53]. This boost signal is also produced by other pathways, such as that promoted by EGFR, HER2, Ras, and Rho, which lead to Stat3 activation [46].

DOI: http://dx.doi.org/10.5772/intechopen.104102

On the other hand, IL-6-induced activation of Stat3 in tumor and stromal cells protects neoplastic cells from the immune surveillance system. This pathway promotes immune evasion [54], by modulating the secretion of various inflammatory factors such as IL-6 and TNF-α [55] and reducing natural killer cell activity [56, 57]. This favors tumor expansion by avoiding immunological control.

Furthermore, the metastatic process is regulated by Stat3, by controlling the capacity for cell migration and invasion of tissues. On one side, Stat3 acts directly on the promoter of MMP genes [58, 59], increasing their expression and thus the ability of cancer cells to degrade the basement membrane/extracellular matrix. Tumor cells then invade the surrounding ECM by migrating due to the action of RhoA on the cytoskeleton [60] after activation of the Stat3/ROCK-myosin pathway. The cells then spread through the circulatory or lymphatic system, forming metastatic foci in lymph nodes and distant organs.

5. Effect of the IL-6/Jak/Stat pathway on neo-angiogenesis mediators

Several authors show that the Jak/Stat pathway plays an important role in neo-angiogenesis through these growth factors.

5.1 HIF-1α

In a hypoxic environment, the HIF-1α protein is stabilized and its proteasomal degradation rate is reduced by slowing down the protein ubiquitination of HIF-1α and thereby achieving enhanced HIF-1α protein levels [61]. This increases its half-life and the cellular concentration of HIF-1α. The IL-6/Jak/Stat3 pathway mediates in the regulation of this process; in such a way that Stat3 interacts with HIF-1α and with VEGF in order to generate greater tumor vascularization (**Figure 2**).

Similar results are obtained after sustained administration of the constitutively active form of Stat3, which causes an increase in HIF-1α transcription, with the consequent increase in HIF-1α protein levels. Changes in HIF-1α levels are also due to the interaction between this molecule and PIAS [62], a negative regulator of the Jak/Stat pathway. Hypoxia causes the interaction between molecules, promoting the stabilization of HIF-1α and prolonging its half-life.

5.2 VEGF

It is well-known that HIF-1α stimulates vascularization and metastasis upon activation of VEGF expression [63]. But there are evidences that show that Stat3 plays a central role in this response. Thus, Xu et al. [64] shows that in various types of human cancer cell lines Stat3 activation induces HIF-1α and up-regulates VEGF expression, promoting tumor angiogenesis [64]. The inhibition of Stat-1/Stat-3 phosphorylation was accompanied by a decrease in VEGF transcription and secretion due to the direct transcriptional action of the VEGF gene by Stat3 (**Figure 2**). On the other hand, Stat3 cooperates with HIF-1α, binding both simultaneously to the promoter region of the VEGF gene, leading to its maximum transcriptional activation and angiogenesis [65].

This action of Stat3 on the VEGF pathway also affects its VEGF receptor. Thus, it has been seen that indirubin suppressed severely the VEGFR-mediated Jak/Stat3 signaling pathway in prostate tumor cells, affecting angiogenesis and tumor growth [66].

Similarly, in pancreatic cancer cell lines, suppression of VEGFR-2 phosphorylation and Stat3-dependent expression of HIF-1α reduced the expression of the Rho-GTPases RhoC, which is downstream of VEGF signaling. This effect plays a vital role in tumor angiogenesis and metastasis [67] because RhoC plays an essential role in transmitting the VEGF signals downstream to angiogenesis and invasiveness [51].

In addition, inhibition of Stat-1/Stat-3 down-regulates other pro-angiogenic factors, such as eNOS, iNOS, MMP-2, and FGF-2 in HUVEC, associated with reduced capillary sprouting and tumor angiogenesis [68, 69]. These molecular findings, taken to clinical practice, translate into a reduction in cell viability, proliferation, adhesion, migration, and tube formation.

Lymphangiogenesis is carried out in a similar way, observing activation of the IL-6-Jak-Stat3-VEGF-C signaling pathway in the growth and invasion process [70, 71].

5.3 PDGF

On the other hand, other aspects must be taken into account. Thus, in the angiogenesis process, it is necessary to increase the cell population, either proliferating new cells or the chemo-attraction of others (**Figure 2**). To do this, PDGF, a growth factor that stands out for being a potent mitogen and chemoattractant for VSMC, stimulates the phosphorylation of Jak-2 and Stat3 in VSMCs [10, 72, 73] and contributes to PDGF-BB-induced mitogenesis [73] and VSMC motility [72]. In addition, PDGF helps regulate the IL-6/Jak-2/Stat pathway through phosphorylation of SOCS, a natural regulator of Jak, by platelet-derived growth factor receptor tyrosine kinase [64].

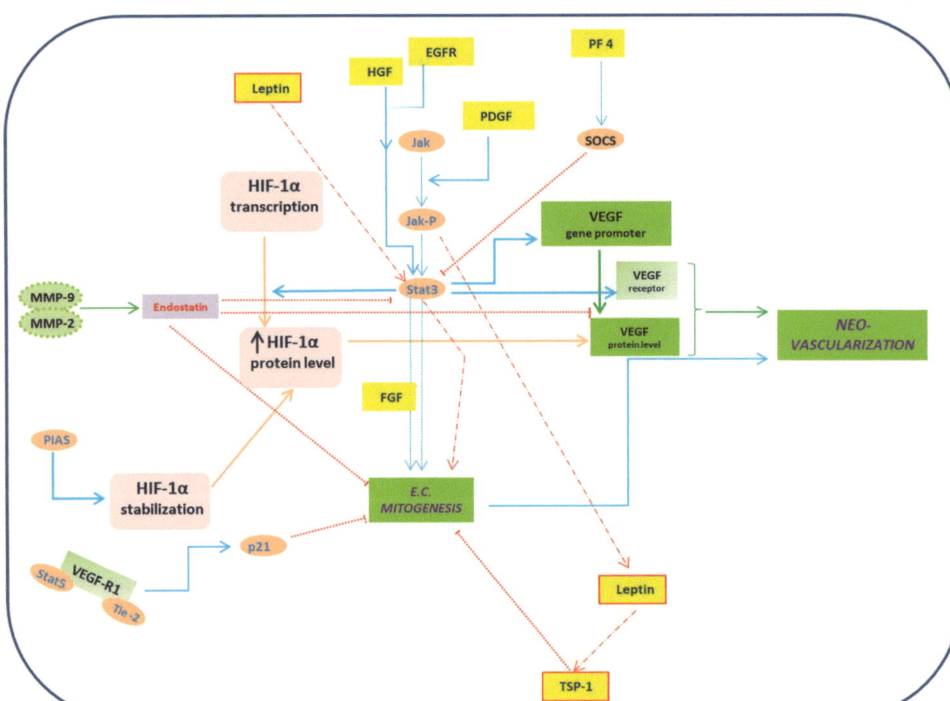

Figure 2.
Diagram that summarizes the neo-angiotizing action of certain cytokines and growth factors that influence neo-angiogenesis and how the mediators of the Jak/Stat pathway act on them.

5.4 FGF

New vessel formation is also regulated by growth factors such as FGF, another downstream effector to IL-6 that induces angiogenic activity in basal cell carcinoma cell lines [74], dependent on the activation of Jak/Stat3. Thus, IL-6 overexpression increases FGF-2 levels (**Figure 2**), tube formation by HUVEC cells, and consequently neoangiogenesis [74].

5.5 Angiopoietins

These molecules are also involved in relevant functions during neo-angiogenesis, such as vascular repair after binding with the endothelial cell-surface receptor tyrosine kinase, Tie2. It also highlights the regulatory activity of Stat on the cell survival, migration, and proliferation [75, 76] by Ang1/Ang2-Tie2 receptor activated. Thus, after Stat5, VEGFR-1 the Tie-2 receptor co-expressed, an increased expression of the cell cycle inhibitor p21 is induced [76], which will arrest cell proliferation (**Figure 2**). On the other hand, angiopoietin-like 4 stimulates Stat 3-mediated iNOS expression and enhances angiogenesis [77].

5.6 HGF

The IL-6/Jak/Stat signaling pathway is regulated by HGF, mediated by SOCS1 [78]. In the case of SOCS3 [79], it counteracted Stat3-dependent keratinocyte migration after being stimulated by HGF (**Figure 2**). In the case of EGFR, SOCS3 is involved in the regulation of IL-6/Jak/Stat signaling, attenuating the EGF signal [78, 80].

5.7 Endostatin

Endostatin activation in the extra cellular environment is enhanced by means of MMP-2/MMP-9 activation, which is accompanied by decreased tumor vascularization [81]. The administration of IL-35 to fibroblast-like synoviocytes produces an inhibition of vascularization due to an increase in the expression of endostatin and a decrease in the expression of VEGF, FGF-2, TNF-α, and IL-6, by means of Stat1 [82]. Synergism between endostatin and Stat3 suppression by a Stat3-siRNA has been observed. In the hepatocarcinoma model, each of both treatments had a potent antitumor effect; but, the combination had a superior effect. It was observed a decreased VEGF expression, decreased cell proliferation, induced cell apoptosis, and inhibited angiogenesis [83] (**Figure 2**).

5.8 PF4

PF4 may contribute to suppress tumor growth in the melanoma murine model, decreasing IL-17, IL-6, and p-Stat3 pathway (**Figure 2**) via up-regulation of SOCS3 expression [84].

5.9 Leptin

Leptin secreted by adipose tissue has a well-known paracrine effect on endothelial, stromal, and tumor cells, enhancing the aggressive tumor behavior. On adipose-derived stromal cells, VEGFA, MMP-2, MMP-9, IGF-1, and b-FGF genes expression are up-regulated and angiogenesis is stimulated by the Jak/Stat3 pathway [85]. In addition, leptin increases the migration and proliferation of VSMC [86, 87], by inducing the phosphorylation of the tyrosine residue of Jak and the activation of its effectors Stat3 and MAPK [88, 89] (**Figure 2**). Jak, on the other hand, produces leptin-dependent up-regulation of TSP-1 [90].

6. Effect of the estrogens on neoangiogenesis mediators

Sex steroids cooperate with the pro- and anti-angiogenic factors involved in the tumor neo-vascularization process. The connection between the inflammatory pathway represented by the IL-6/Jak-Stat pathway, and the tumor estrogenic pathway is very close and is involved in the pathogenic processes of these diseases [43].

Recently, evidence has emerged showing that cytokines generated during the inflammatory process interact with estrogen signaling pathways [43]. On one side, there is a very close relationship between ER α protein levels and Stat 1 activity (**Figure 3**). Thus, if Stat1 levels are insufficient or its function is blocked, a decrease in ERα levels and cell proliferation is observed. This occurs through the direct action of Stat1 on the promoter region of ERα, regulating the transcription of mRNA levels [91].

On the other hand, estrogenic activity has been found in adipose tissue and tumoral stroma. Thus, immunohistochemical studies have found the expression of cytochrome P450 aromatase, responsible for the aromatization of adrenal and testicular androgens into estrogens (**Figure 3**). It is also known that the IL-6/Jak/Stat pathway stimulates the cytochrome P450 aromatase expression, transforming tissue androgens into estrogens that will act in a paracrine manner on the tumor, causing tumor growth and development [92].

This connection between IL-6/Jak/Stat and estrogens is regulated, in such a way that there is negative regulation of Jak2 with respect to ERα [43] because Jak2 induces

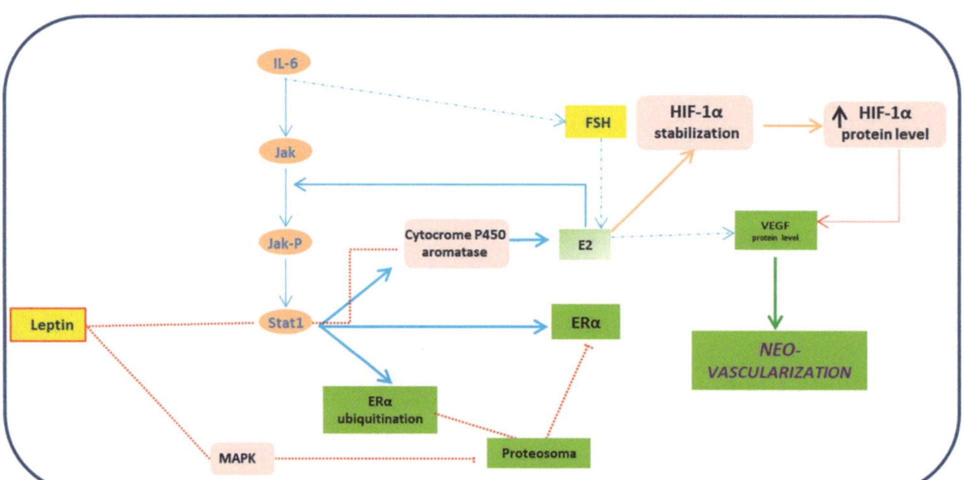

Figure 3.
Diagram summarizing the action of how estrogens and mediators of the Jak/Stat pathway interact during the process of neo-angiogenesis.

the ubiquitination of ERα for being degraded in the proteasome (**Figure 3**). On the other hand, sustained treatment with E2 induces Jak-2 expression, thus controlling the formation and destruction of these molecules.

These observations are integrated by the adipose tissue cytokine leptin function. It activates the phosphorylation of the tyrosine residue of the receptor and causes the activation of its effectors Stat3 and MAPK (**Figure 3**). In this way, the estrogenic pathway is enhanced at the tissue level, since Stat3 induces the generation of estrogens by aromatization of androgens, and MAPK stops the proteasomal degradation of ERα [93], enhancing the estrogenic status [43].

Estrogens, in addition to synergizing with the IL-6/Jak/Stat pathway, regulate the action of mediators involved in the neo-angiogenesis process (**Figure 3**). Thus, regarding HIF-1α, estrogens stabilize the protein in normoxia by regulating its expression through the Akt pathway [63, 94].

In addition, IL-6 induces the expression of VEGF in granulosa cells through FSH mediation, favoring the expression of HIF-1α and COX2, thanks to the activation of the Jak/Stat3 pathway (**Figure 3**). Other evidence indicates that ovarian steroids increase the production of HGF by peritoneal macrophages, promoting the proliferation of endothelial cells and the organization of capillaries.

The angiopoietins, promote the formation of endothelial cells through the mediation of estrogens. Thus, the up-regulation of brain Ang-1 mRNA caused an increase in the capillary density. Besides, E2 acting through ERβ up-regulates Ang-2, increased Tie-2 phosphorylation, and promoted angiogenesis [95].

In ER-positive breast cancer tumor cells, estrogens control the production of TSP-1, which is under the direct control of estrogens, performing regulatory functions favorable to tumor growth [96].

It is also the case that a growth factor is influenced by both pathways. In the case of FGF, while estrogens potentiate its release, it signaling pathway was mediated by activated Stat1 [97].

All these coordinated measures between both systems are aimed at enhancing vascular neo-formation and thus potential metastatic dissemination.

Conflict of interest

"The authors declare no conflict of interest."

Authorship

José Manuel García-Castellano (JMGC); David García-Padrón (DGP); Nerea Martínez-Aragón (NMA); Margarita Ramírez-Sánchez (MRS); Vicente Vera-Gutiérrez (VVG); Leandro Fernández-Pérez (LFP).

- Substantially contribute to the conception or design of the work; or the acquisition, analysis, or interpretation of data for the work: JMGC, LFP

- Participate in drafting or revising the work: DGP, NMA, MRS, VVG

- Approve the final version of the work to be published: JMGC, LFP, DGP, NMA, MRS, VVG

Author details

José Manuel García-Castellano[1,2,3,4*], David García-Padrón[2†], Nerea Martínez-Aragón[2†], Margarita Ramírez-Sánchez[5], Vicente Vera-Gutiérrez[6] and Leandro Fernández-Pérez[7]

1 Orthopedic Surgery and Traumatology, Maternal and Child University Hospital Complex of Gran Canaria, Las Palmas de Gran Canaria, Canary Islands, Spain

2 Molecular Oncology Laboratory, Research Unit, Maternal and Child University Hospital Complex of Gran Canaria, Las Palmas de Gran Canaria, Canary Islands, Spain

3 Department of Medical and Surgical Sciences, University Institute of Biomedical and Health Research (IUIBS), University of Las Palmas de Gran Canaria, Spain

4 Spanish Sarcoma Research Group (GEIS), Spain

5 Physical Medicine and Rehabilitation Service, University Hospital of Gran Canaria Doctor Negrín, Las Palmas de Gran Canaria, Spain

6 Orthopedic Surgery and Traumatology, University Hospital of Gran Canaria Doctor Negrín, Las Palmas de Gran Canaria, Spain

7 Faculty of Health Sciences, Department of Clinical Sciences, Laboratory of Pharmacology, University of Las Palmas de Gran Canaria, Spain

*Address all correspondence to: jmgc_61@yahoo.com

† Both authors contributed equally to this work.

References

[1] Semenza GL. The hypoxic tumor microenvironment: A driving force for breast cancer progression. Biochimica et Biophysica Acta. 2016;**1863**(3):382-391

[2] Vaupel P. Hypoxia and aggressive tumor phenotype: Implications for therapy and prognosis. The Oncologist. 2008;**13**(Suppl. 3):21-26

[3] Vaupel P. The role of hypoxia-induced factors in tumor progression. The Oncologist. 2004;**9**(Suppl. 5):10-17

[4] Höckel M, Vaupel P. Tumor hypoxia: Definitions and current clinical, biologic, and molecular aspects. Journal of the National Cancer Institute. 2001;**93**(4):266-276

[5] Brown JM. Tumor hypoxia in cancer therapy. Methods in Enzymology. 2007;**435**:297-321

[6] Zhou J et al. Tumor hypoxia and cancer progression. Cancer Letters. 2006;**237**(1):10-21

[7] Kim JW, Gao P, Dang CV. Effects of hypoxia on tumor metabolism. Cancer Metastasis Reviews. 2007;**26**(2):291-298

[8] Teleanu RI, Chircov C. Tumor angiogenesis and anti-angiogenic strategies for cancer treatment. Journal of Clinical Medicine. 2019;**9**(1):84

[9] Repsold L et al. An overview of the role of platelets in angiogenesis, apoptosis and autophagy in chronic myeloid leukaemia. Cancer Cell International. 2017;**17**(1):89

[10] Wojtukiewicz MZ et al. Platelets and cancer angiogenesis nexus. Cancer Metastasis Reviews. 2017;**36**(2): 249-262

[11] Rust R, Gantner C, Schwab ME. Pro- and antiangiogenic therapies: Current status and clinical implications. The FASEB Journal. 2019;**33**(1):34-48

[12] Mazurek R et al. Vascular cells in blood vessel wall development and disease. Advances in Pharmacology. 2017;**78**:323-350

[13] Ferrara N, Gerber HP, LeCouter J. The biology of VEGF and its receptors. Nature Medicine. 2003;**9**(6):669-676

[14] Duran CL et al. Molecular regulation of sprouting angiogenesis. Comprehensive Physiology. 2017;**8**(1):153-235

[15] Jain RK. Molecular regulation of vessel maturation. Nature Medicine. 2003;**9**(6):685-693

[16] Semenza GL. HIF-1: Mediator of physiological and pathophysiological responses to hypoxia. Journal of Applied Physiology. 2000;**88**(4):1474-1480

[17] Zhong H et al. Overexpression of hypoxia-inducible factor 1alpha in common human cancers and their metastases. Cancer Research. 1999;**59**(22):5830-5835

[18] Folkman J. Angiogenesis: An organizing principle for drug discovery? Nature Reviews. Drug Discovery. 2007;**6**(4):273-286

[19] Henning RJ. Therapeutic angiogenesis: Angiogenic growth factors for ischemic heart disease. Future Cardiology. 2016;**12**(5):585-599

[20] Raica M, Cimpean AM. Platelet-derived growth factor (PDGF)/PDGF receptors (PDGFR) Axis as target

for antitumor and antiangiogenic therapy. Pharmaceuticals (Basel). 2010;**3**(3):572-599

[21] Yu J, Ustach C, Kim HR. Platelet-derived growth factor signaling and human cancer. Journal of Biochemistry and Molecular Biology. 2003;**36**(1):49-59

[22] Yu X, Ye F. Role of angiopoietins in development of cancer and neoplasia associated with viral infection. Cell. 2020;**9**(2):457

[23] Xue F et al. Hepatocyte growth factor gene therapy accelerates regeneration in cirrhotic mouse livers after hepatectomy. Gut. 2003;**52**(5):694-700

[24] Funakoshi H, Nakamura T. Hepatocyte growth factor: From diagnosis to clinical applications. Clinica Chimica Acta. 2003;**327**(1-2):1-23

[25] Stuart KA et al. Hepatocyte growth factor/scatter factor-induced intracellular signalling. International Journal of Experimental Pathology. 2000;**81**(1):17-30

[26] Kanno Y. The role of fibrinolytic regulators in vascular dysfunction of systemic sclerosis. International Journal of Molecular Sciences. 2019;**20**(3):619

[27] Tanabe K, Sato Y, Wada J. Endogenous antiangiogenic factors in chronic kidney disease: Potential biomarkers of progression. International Journal of Molecular Sciences. 2018;**19**(7):1859

[28] Poluzzi C, Iozzo RV, Schaefer L. Endostatin and endorepellin: A common route of action for similar angiostatic cancer avengers. Advanced Drug Delivery Reviews. 2016;**97**:156-173

[29] Olver TD, Ferguson BS, Laughlin MH. Molecular mechanisms for exercise training-induced changes in vascular structure and function: Skeletal muscle, cardiac muscle, and the brain. Progress in Molecular Biology and Translational Science. 2015;**135**:227-257

[30] Lawler PR, Lawler J. Molecular basis for the regulation of angiogenesis by thrombospondin-1 and -2. Cold Spring Harbor Perspectives in Medicine. 2012;**2**(5):a006627

[31] Semenza GL. HIF-1 and human disease: One highly involved factor. Genes & Development. 2000;**14**(16):1983-1991

[32] Semenza GL. Targeting HIF-1 for cancer therapy. Nature Reviews. Cancer. 2003;**3**(10):721-732

[33] Zimna A, Kurpisz M. Hypoxia-inducible Factor-1 in physiological and pathophysiological angiogenesis: Applications and therapies. BioMed Research International. 2015;**2015**:549412

[34] Wang GL et al. Hypoxia-inducible factor 1 is a basic-helix-loop-helix-PAS heterodimer regulated by cellular O2 tension. Proceedings of the National Academy of Sciences of the United States of America. 1995;**92**(12):5510-5514

[35] Carmeliet P et al. Role of HIF-1alpha in hypoxia-mediated apoptosis, cell proliferation and tumour angiogenesis. Nature. 1998;**394**(6692):485-490

[36] Schofield CJ, Ratcliffe PJ. Oxygen sensing by HIF hydroxylases. Nature Reviews. Molecular Cell Biology. 2004;**5**(5):343-354

[37] Gruber M, Simon MC. Hypoxia-inducible factors, hypoxia, and tumor angiogenesis. Current Opinion in Hematology. 2006;**13**(3):169-174

[38] Pouysségur J, Dayan F, Mazure NM. Hypoxia signalling in cancer and

approaches to enforce tumour regression. Nature. 2006;**441**(7092):437-443

[39] Jaakkola P et al. Targeting of HIF-alpha to the von Hippel-Lindau ubiquitylation complex by O2-regulated prolyl hydroxylation. Science. 2001; **292**(5516):468-472

[40] Semenza GL. Targeting hypoxia-inducible factor 1 to stimulate tissue vascularization. Journal of Investigative Medicine. 2016;**64**(2):361-363

[41] Inampudi C et al. Angiogenesis in peripheral arterial disease. Current Opinion in Pharmacology. 2018;**39**:60-67

[42] Buchert M, Burns CJ, Ernst M. Targeting JAK kinase in solid tumors: Emerging opportunities and challenges. Oncogene. 2016;**35**(8):939-951

[43] Gupta N, Mayer D. Interaction of JAK with steroid receptor function. Jakstat. 2013;**2**(4):e24911

[44] Lee H et al. Persistently activated Stat3 maintains constitutive NF-kappaB activity in tumors. Cancer Cell. 2009;**15**(4):283-293

[45] Yu H, Pardoll D, Jove R. STATs in cancer inflammation and immunity: A leading role for STAT3. Nature Reviews. Cancer. 2009;**9**(11):798-809

[46] Bournazou E, Bromberg J. Targeting the tumor microenvironment: JAK-STAT3 signaling. Jakstat. 2013;**2**(2):e23828

[47] Zhuang G et al. Tumour-secreted miR-9 promotes endothelial cell migration and angiogenesis by activating the JAK-STAT pathway. The EMBO Journal. 2012;**31**(17):3513-3523

[48] Bartoli M et al. VEGF differentially activates STAT3 in microvascular endothelial cells. The FASEB Journal. 2003;**17**(11):1562-1564

[49] Leong H, Mathur PS, Greene GL. Green tea catechins inhibit angiogenesis through suppression of STAT3 activation. Breast Cancer Research and Treatment. 2009;**117**(3):505-515

[50] Dong Y et al. Cucurbitacin E, a tetracyclic triterpenes compound from Chinese medicine, inhibits tumor angiogenesis through VEGFR2-mediated Jak2-STAT3 signaling pathway. Carcinogenesis. 2010;**31**(12):2097-2104

[51] Lincoln DW, Phillips PG, Bove K. Estrogen-induced Ets-1 promotes capillary formation in an in vitro tumor angiogenesis model. Breast Cancer Research and Treatment. 2003;**78**(2):167-178

[52] Banerjee K, Resat H. Constitutive activation of STAT3 in breast cancer cells: A review. International Journal of Cancer. 2016;**138**(11):2570-2578

[53] Liu Q et al. IL-6 promotion of glioblastoma cell invasion and angiogenesis in U251 and T98G cell lines. Journal of Neuro-Oncology. 2010;**100**(2):165-176

[54] Xin H et al. Antiangiogenic and antimetastatic activity of JAK inhibitor AZD1480. Cancer Research. 2011;**71**(21):6601-6610

[55] Nguyen DX, Bos PD, Massagué J. Metastasis: From dissemination to organ-specific colonization. Nature Reviews. Cancer. 2009;**9**(4):274-284

[56] Wang T et al. Regulation of the innate and adaptive immune responses by Stat-3 signaling in tumor cells. Nature Medicine. 2004;**10**(1):48-54

[57] Giraud S et al. Functional interaction of STAT3 transcription factor with

the coactivator NcoA/SRC1a. The Journal of Biological Chemistry. 2002;**277**(10):8004-8011

[58] Xie TX et al. Stat3 activation regulates the expression of matrix metalloproteinase-2 and tumor invasion and metastasis. Oncogene. 2004;**23**(20):3550-3560

[59] Itoh M et al. Requirement of STAT3 activation for maximal collagenase-1 (MMP-1) induction by epidermal growth factor and malignant characteristics in T24 bladder cancer cells. Oncogene. 2006;**25**(8):1195-1204

[60] Pan YR et al. STAT3-coordinated migration facilitates the dissemination of diffuse large B-cell lymphomas. Nature Communications. 2018;**9**(1):3696

[61] Jung JE et al. STAT3 inhibits the degradation of HIF-1alpha by pVHL-mediated ubiquitination. Experimental & Molecular Medicine. 2008;**40**(5):479-485

[62] Shuai K, Liu B. Regulation of gene-activation pathways by PIAS proteins in the immune system. Nature Reviews. Immunology. 2005;**5**(8):593-605

[63] Dey P et al. Estrogen receptor β2 induces hypoxia signature of gene expression by stabilizing HIF-1α in prostate cancer. PLoS One. 2015;**10**(5):e0128239

[64] Sommer U et al. Mechanisms of SOCS3 phosphorylation upon interleukin-6 stimulation. Contributions of Src- and receptor-tyrosine kinases. The Journal of Biological Chemistry. 2005;**280**(36):31478-31488

[65] Oh MK et al. Hypoxia-inducible factor-1alpha enhances haptoglobin gene expression by improving binding of STAT3 to the promoter. The Journal of Biological Chemistry. 2011;**286**(11): 8857-8865

[66] Chen SH et al. Activated STAT3 is a mediator and biomarker of VEGF endothelial activation. Cancer Biology & Therapy. 2008;**7**(12):1994-2003

[67] Boreddy SR, Sahu RP, Srivastava SK. Benzyl isothiocyanate suppresses pancreatic tumor angiogenesis and invasion by inhibiting HIF-α/VEGF/rho-GTPases: Pivotal role of STAT-3. PLoS One. 2011;**6**(10):e25799

[68] Li S et al. Icaritin inhibits JAK/STAT3 signaling and growth of renal cell carcinoma. PLoS One. 2013;**8**(12):e81657

[69] Bhat TA et al. Acacetin inhibits in vitro and in vivo angiogenesis and downregulates Stat signaling and VEGF expression. Cancer Prevention Research (Philadelphia, PA). 2013;**6**(10):1128-1139

[70] Zhao G et al. IL-6 mediates the signal pathway of JAK-STAT3-VEGF-C promoting growth, invasion and lymphangiogenesis in gastric cancer. Oncology Reports. 2016;**35**(3):1787-1795

[71] Nielsen SR et al. IL-27 inhibits lymphatic endothelial cell proliferation by STAT1-regulated gene expression. Microcirculation. 2013;**20**(6):555-564

[72] Neeli I et al. An essential role of the Jak-2/STAT-3/cytosolic phospholipase A(2) axis in platelet-derived growth factor BB-induced vascular smooth muscle cell motility. The Journal of Biological Chemistry. 2004;**279**(44):46122-46128

[73] Simon AR et al. Role of the JAK-STAT pathway in PDGF-stimulated proliferation of human airway smooth muscle cells. American Journal of Physiology. Lung Cellular and Molecular Physiology. 2002;**282**(6):L1296-L1304

[74] Jee SH et al. Interleukin-6 induced basic fibroblast growth factor-dependent angiogenesis in basal cell carcinoma cell line via JAK/STAT3 and PI3-kinase/Akt pathways. The Journal of Investigative Dermatology. 2004;**123**(6):1169-1175

[75] Loughna S, Sato TN. Angiopoietin and Tie signaling pathways in vascular development. Matrix Biology. 2001;**20**(5-6):319-325

[76] Korpelainen EI et al. Endothelial receptor tyrosine kinases activate the STAT signaling pathway: Mutant Tie-2 causing venous malformations signals a distinct STAT activation response. Oncogene. 1999;**18**(1):1-8

[77] Chong HC et al. Angiopoietin-like 4 stimulates STAT3-mediated iNOS expression and enhances angiogenesis to accelerate wound healing in diabetic mice. Molecular Therapy. 2014;**22**(9):1593-1604

[78] Khan MGM et al. Hepatocyte growth control by SOCS1 and SOCS3. Cytokine. 2019;**121**:154733

[79] Garajová I et al. c-met as a target for personalized therapy. Translational Oncogenomics. 2015;7(Suppl. 1):13-31

[80] Eitsuka T et al. Synergistic anticancer effect of tocotrienol combined with chemotherapeutic agents or dietary components: A review. International Journal of Molecular Sciences. 2016;**17**(10):1605

[81] Nilsson UW, Dabrosin C. Estradiol and tamoxifen regulate endostatin generation via matrix metalloproteinase activity in breast cancer in vivo. Cancer Research. 2006;**66**(9):4789-4794

[82] Wu S et al. Interleukin-35 inhibits angiogenesis through STAT1 signalling in rheumatoid synoviocytes. Clinical and Experimental Rheumatology. 2018;**36**(2):223-227

[83] Jia H et al. Antitumor effects of Stat3-siRNA and endostatin combined therapies, delivered by attenuated Salmonella, on orthotopically implanted hepatocarcinoma. Cancer Immunology, Immunotherapy. 2012;**61**(11):1977-1987

[84] Fang S et al. Platelet factor 4 inhibits IL-17/Stat3 pathway via upregulation of SOCS3 expression in melanoma. Inflammation. 2014;**37**(5):1744-1750

[85] Xue C et al. The JAK/STAT3 signalling pathway regulated angiogenesis in an endothelial cell/adipose-derived stromal cell co-culture, 3D gel model. Cell Proliferation, 2017;**50**(1):e12307

[86] Li L et al. Signaling pathways involved in human vascular smooth muscle cell proliferation and matrix metalloproteinase-2 expression induced by leptin: Inhibitory effect of metformin. Diabetes. 2005;**54**(7):2227-2234

[87] Oda A, Taniguchi T, Yokoyama M. Leptin stimulates rat aortic smooth muscle cell proliferation and migration. The Kobe Journal of Medical Sciences. 2001;**47**(3):141-150

[88] Frühbeck G. Intracellular signalling pathways activated by leptin. The Biochemical Journal. 2006;**393**(Pt 1):7-20

[89] Hegyi K et al. Leptin-induced signal transduction pathways. Cell Biology International. 2004;**28**(3):159-169

[90] Chavez RJ et al. Upregulation of thrombospondin-1 expression by leptin in vascular smooth muscle cells via JAK2- and MAPK-dependent pathways. American Journal of Physiology. Cell Physiology. 2012;**303**(2):C179-C191

[91] Hu Q et al. SOCS1 silencing can break high-dose dendritic cell immunotherapy-induced immune tolerance. Molecular Medicine Reports. 2008;**1**(1):61-70

[92] Zhao Y et al. Aromatase P450 gene expression in human adipose tissue. Role of a Jak/STAT pathway in regulation of the adipose-specific promoter. The Journal of Biological Chemistry. 1995;**270**(27):16449-16457

[93] Andò S, Catalano S. The multifactorial role of leptin in driving the breast cancer microenvironment. Nature Reviews. Endocrinology. 2011;**8**(5):263-275

[94] Hua K et al. Estrogen and progestin regulate HIF-1alpha expression in ovarian cancer cell lines via the activation of Akt signaling transduction pathway. Oncology Reports. 2009;**21**(4):893-898

[95] Gu J et al. Targeting the ERβ/Angiopoietin-2/Tie-2 signaling-mediated angiogenesis with the FDA-approved anti-estrogen Faslodex to increase the Sunitinib sensitivity in RCC. Cell Death & Disease. 2020;**11**(5):367

[96] Hyder SM, Liang Y, Wu J. Estrogen regulation of thrombospondin-1 in human breast cancer cells. International Journal of Cancer. 2009;**125**(5):1045-1053

[97] Mossahebi-Mohammadi M et al. FGF signaling pathway: A key regulator of stem cell pluripotency. Frontiers in Cell and Development Biology. 2020;**8**:79

Chapter 5

Modulators of Tumor Angiogenesis: Insights into the Role of Galectin-3 and IL-17 Signaling

Gordana D. Radosavljevic, Jelena Pantic, Bojana Simovic Markovic and Nebojsa Arsenijevic

Abstract

Angiogenesis is a pivotal point in tumor progression driven by firmly orchestrated process of forming the new blood vessels relying on the complex signaling network. Here, the pleiotropic functions of Galectin-3 and IL-17 in tumor progression have been overviewed through their impacts on angiogenesis. As a key player in tumor microenvironment, Galectin-3 orchestrates practically all critical events during angiogenic cascade through interaction with various ligands and their downstream signaling pathways. Galectin-3 shapes chronic inflammatory tumor microenvironment that is closely related to angiogenesis by sharing common signaling cascades and molecules. In chronic inflammatory makeup of tumor microenvironment, IL-17 contributes to tumorigenesis and progression *via* promoting critical events such as angiogenesis and creation of immunosuppressive milieu. VEGF, as the master regulator of tumor angiogenesis, is the main target of Galectin-3 and IL-17 action. The better understanding of Galectin-3 and IL-17 in tumor biology will undoubtedly contribute to controlling tumor progression. Therefore, as important modulators of tumor angiogenesis, Galectin-3 and IL-17 may be perceived as the potential therapeutic targets in tumor including anti-angiogenic therapy.

Keywords: galectin-3, IL-17, VEGF, tumor angiogenesis, tumor progression

1. Introduction

Tumor angiogenesis or aberrant vascularization is considered a critical hallmark of tumor progression that is inevitable for tumor growth and metastatic spread [1]. This complex multistep process of new vasculature formation from pre-existing blood vessels is triggered by numerous signals from tumor cells in a phase of rapid growth [1]. The expression and secretion of various activators and inhibitors of angiogenesis are regulated by gene mutation (e.g., oncogenes and tumor-suppressor genes), and microenvironmental factors such as hypoxia and accumulation of different metabolites [2, 3]. As the growing tumor requires more blood vessels for nutrition and oxygen supply, angiogenic pathways are induced by tilting the balance toward pro-angiogenic molecules (angiogenic switch) to drive new blood vessel growth [3].

IntechOpen

High expression levels of pro-angiogenic factors reflect the tumor aggressiveness [4]. Within the angiogenic cascade, a diverse group of mediators are shown in **Figure 1**. These molecules participate in the establishment of new tumor vessels in various ways. Among them, vascular endothelial growth factor (VEGF), also called VEGF-A, is key "molecular player" that modifies the endothelial barriers [3]. Moreover, VEGF as master regulator of angiogenesis in tumor tissues and its receptors, particularly VEGFR-2, have been implicated in tumor vascularization [3]. Namely, activation of VEGF/VEGFR-2 signaling pathways triggers an angiogenic program in the endothelial cells (ECs) [3]. Thus, VEGF binds to its cognate receptor that results in autophosphorylation of specific tyrosine residues of VEGFR-2, and consequential activation of multiple downstream signaling networks in the vascular endothelial cells through the recruiting of the MAP kinase (ERK1/2 and p38), PI3K, AKT, PLC-γ, and JAK-STAT [5–7]. The final result is the activation of full range of

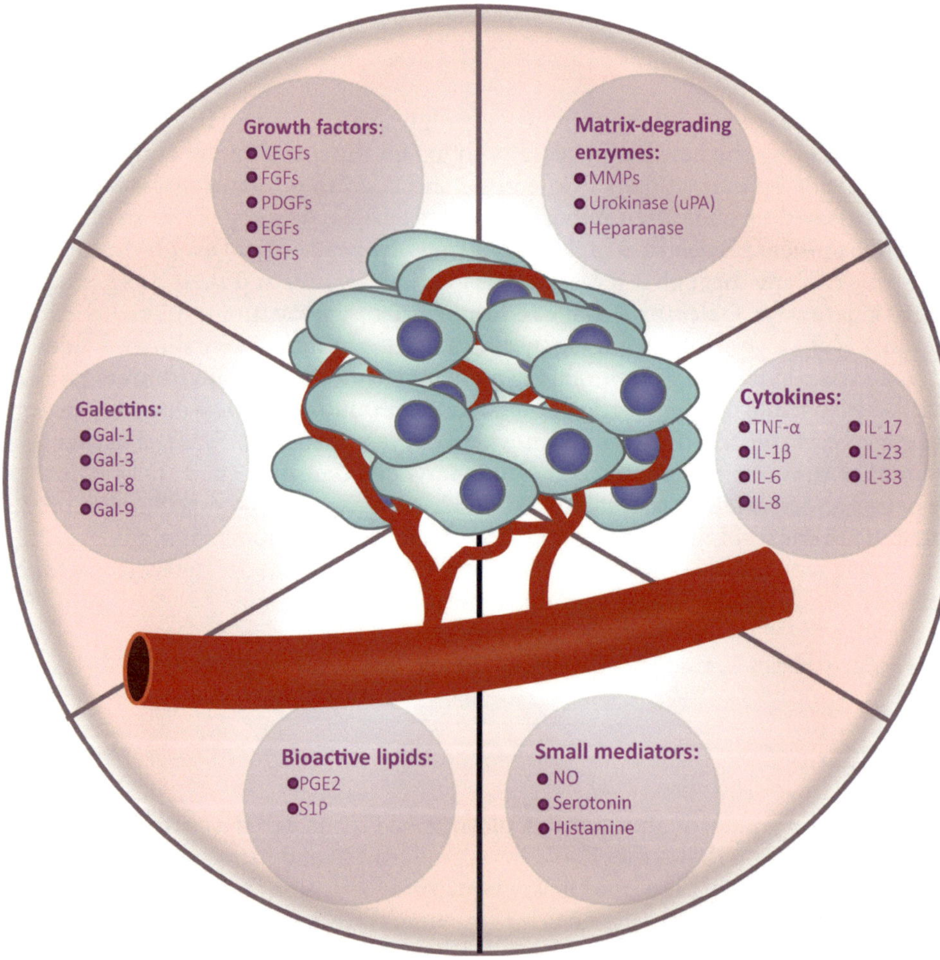

Figure 1.
Pro-angiogenic mediators implicated in the tumor angiogenesis. Plethora of mediators that promotes tumor angiogenesis can be categorized into several groups. VEGFs-vascular endothelial factors; FGFs-fibroblast growth factors; PDGFs-platelet-derived growth factor; EGFs-epidermal growth factor; TGFs-transforming growth factors; MMPs-matrix metalloproteinases; uPA-urokinase-type plasminogen activator; TNF-α-tumor necrosis factor-α; NO-nitric oxide; PGE2-prostaglandin E2; S1P-sphingosine-1-phosphate.

biological responses that modulate angiogenesis, including vascular permeability as well as endothelial cell proliferation, survival, adhesion, and migration.

It is well established that VEGF is multifunctional molecule. VEGF has been first identified as vascular permeability factor, which exerts potent ability to increase vascular permeability, resulting in leakage of plasma protein and other molecules out of blood vessels [8]. Furthermore, VEGF is a potent mitogen that is highly specific for ECs and stimulates cell proliferation through VEGFR-2-mediated activation of the RAS/RAF/ERK/MAPK pathway [9]. Acting as survival factor for ECs, VEGF increases expression of the anti-apoptotic proteins Bcl-2 and A1 in the ECs [10]. On the other hand, VEGF also participates in tumor angiogenesis through increased migration and invasion of ECs by enhancing of matrix metalloproteinases (MMPs) release [3], and further amplifying angiogenesis by enhanced recruitment and homing of bone marrow derived vascular precursor cells [11]. PI3K/AKT signaling promotes VEGF-mediated invasion and metastasis of ECs [12].

VEGF expression is tightly regulated by plethora of transcriptional regulators, such as transcription factor called hypoxia-inducible factor (HIF). Beside them, VEGF signaling is also upregulated by multiple stimuli, including cytokines and galectins by tumor microenvironments. We discuss the role of IL-17 and Galectin-3 in mediating angiogenesis, either directly or indirectly *via* induction of pro-angiogenic factors such as VEGF. The better understanding of Galectin-3 and IL-17 in tumor biology will undoubtedly contribute to controlling tumor progression. Namely, we will review the role of these two molecules in tumor angiogenesis and highlight the other mechanisms involved in the acceleration of tumor growth and metastases.

2. Galectin-3 and IL-17: an important piece in the puzzle of tumor microenvironment

The tumor microenvironment represents a complex ecosystem involving interactions between tumor cells, ECs, epithelial cells, immune cells, fibroblasts, and the extracellular matrix, as well as secreted cytokines and growth factors. All of these factors provide essential support for the tumor progression. The dynamic cross-talk between angiogenesis and tumor microenvironment is important to further accelerate tumor growth and metastasis [13]. Thus, released angiogenic factors can promote tumor immunosuppression by inhibiting maturation of dendritic cells, increasing mobilization of immunosuppressive cells, and suppressing CD8 + T cell activity [14]. The tumor microenvironment, in turn, produces numerous soluble molecules and growth factors that stimulate angiogenesis, thus forming a vicious circle for tumor progression [15]. Increasing evidence suggests that Galectin-3 and IL-17 are the significant pieces of that puzzle that shape angiogenesis and tumor progression in many ways (**Figure 2**).

Galectin-3, a unique chimaera-type member of the lectin family with selectivity for β-galactosides, is a versatile galectin involved in fundamental biological processes as well as various pathological circumstances [16, 17]. This evolutionary conserved molecule is usually overexpressed in variety types of tumor [18]. The ECs, immune cells, mesenchymal stem cells (MSCs), cancer-associated fibroblasts (CAFs), and myofibroblasts also produce and secrete Galectin-3 [19–21]. Galectin-3 expression is higher in endothelial progenitor cells as compared with normal ECs [22]. However, the tumor microenvironment, for example, tumor cells, inflammatory cells, and/or

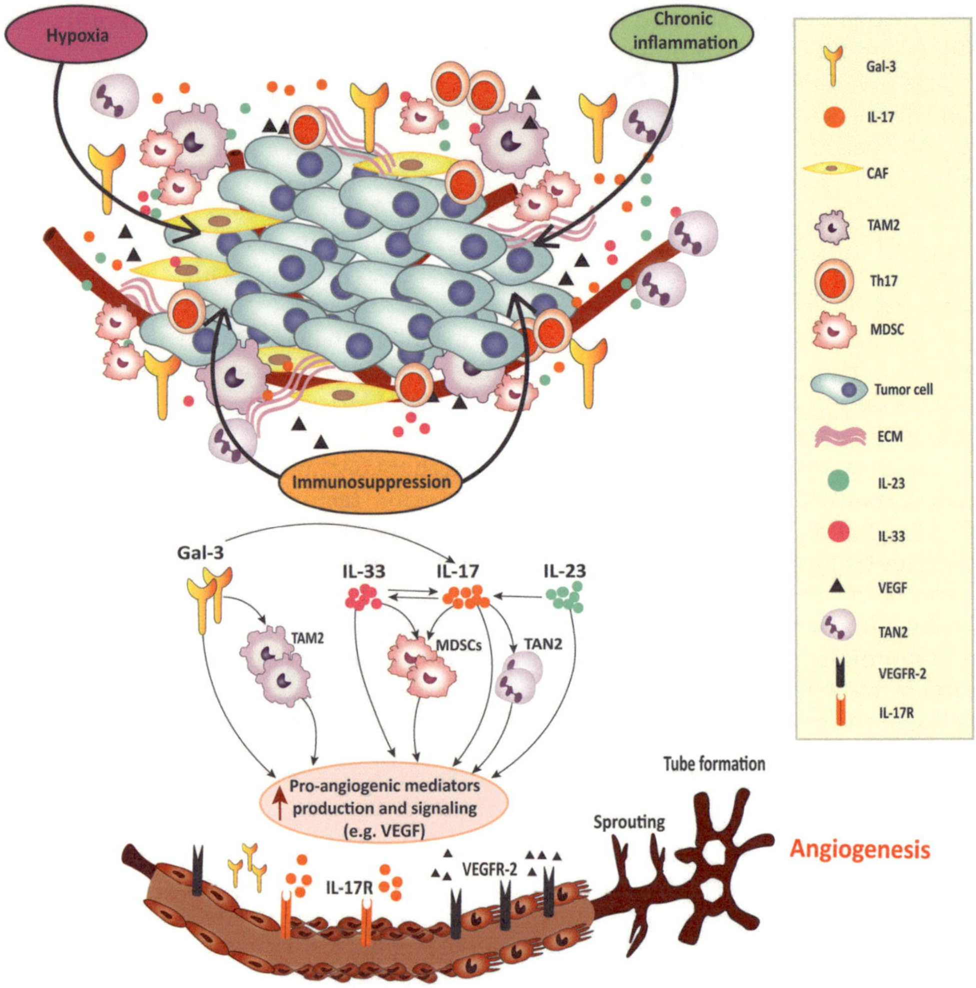

Figure 2.
Pro-angiogenic effects of Galectin-3 and IL-17 as a part of tumor progression machinery. Many cells and soluble mediators create tumor microenvironment characterized by hypoxia, chronic inflammation, and immunosuppression. Galectin-3 participates in all steps of angiogenic cascade via activation of different signaling pathways and/or polarization of macrophages toward pro-tumorigenic TAM2 phenotype. Galectin-3 affects the production of pro-inflammatory cytokines implicated in tumor promotion. Within the complex cytokine network in tumor microenvironment, IL-17 is recognized as one of the critical stimulators of the production of pro-angiogenic mediators, including VEGF. IL-17 mediates the recruitment of TAN2 thus augmenting angiogenic factors release. IL-23 and IL-33 seem to be significant co-workers in triggering angiogenic cascade. Both IL-17 and IL-33 induce recruitment of pro-angiogenic MDSC, while IL-23 further promotes function, survival, and expansions of Th17 lymphocytes, and subsequent IL-17 production. The activation, proliferation, and migration of endothelial cells, as well as sprouting and tube formation, precede the formation of new blood vessels critical for tumor progression. CAF-cancer-associated fibroblast; TAM-tumor-associated macrophage; TAN-tumor-associated neutrophil; MDSC-myeloid-derived suppressor cell; ECM-extracellular matrix.

specific glycan-ligands on galectin-binding proteins, alters endothelial Galectin-3 expression as it provide most of the signals to which the ECs respond [23, 24]. Accordingly, pro-inflammatory cytokine IL-1β increases Galectin-3 expression by ECs [25]. ECs not only have a pivotal role in angiogenesis, but also they facilitate tumor invasion by secreting growth factors and extracellular matrix proteinases [26]. Released molecules sequentially increase chances that tumor cells enter to the circulation and metastasis [26].

Depending on cell types and cellular localization, Galectin-3 drives force in the diverse processes critical in tumor biology, including apoptosis, invasion, metastasis, immune surveillance, gene expression, and inflammation [27]. The cytoplasmic Galectin-3 blocks apoptotic machinery in tumor cells [16] through several mechanisms [28]. Galectin-3 secreted by tumor cells contributes to immunosuppression within the tumor microenvironment by polarizing to pro-tumor phenotype of tumor-associated macrophages 2 (TAM2), restricting T cell receptor clustering, and triggering apoptosis of CD8 + T lymphocytes, further facilitating tumor escape [29]. The upregulation of Galectin-3 by TAMs in the hypoxic regions of breast cancer promotes tumor cell migration and invasion and TAMs-mediated metastasis, as well as angiogenesis [30]. Expression of Galectin-3 in CAFs in breast cancer has been associated with distant metastasis [31]. Galectin-3 is also found in extracellular vesicles released by tumor cells, and it seems that this galectin is critical regulator in cell-cell and cell-extracellular matrix interactions [32]. Endothelial Galectin-3 expression in the lungs cooperates with poly-N-acetyl-lactosamine on N-glycans of B16-F1 murine melanoma cells, as a ligand for Galectin-3 [33]. Our data demonstrated that host-derived Galectin-3 facilitates B16-F1 cell adhesion to the metastatic target and interferes with efficiency of the antitumor immune response, thereby accelerating melanoma metastasis [34].

Tumor angiogenesis and chronic inflammation are closely related and often share common signaling pathways and molecules [35]. In addition to angiogenesis, Galectin-3 participates in shaping of tumor inflammatory microenvironment likely through the recruitment of inflammatory cells and modification of their polarization [36], as well as the production of pro-inflammatory cytokines that have been implicated in tumor promotion (**Figure 2**, [37]). Overexpressed pro-inflammatory IL-1, IL-6, and TNF-α contribute to various steps of tumor progression [38]. This cytokine network, required for the establishment of chronic inflammation in the tumor microenvironment, facilitates tumor growth and metastasis, enhances angiogenesis, and inhibits immune surveillance [39]. In particular, tumor-infiltrating Th17 lymphocytes orchestrate the maintenance of chronic inflammation. IL-6, TGF-β, and IL-1β are pivotal drivers of development of Th17 cells that secrete IL-17 and other cytokines. Although IL-23 is not required for triggering Th17 differentiation, it is essential for the function, survival, and expansion of Th17 lymphocytes in the inflamed tissue [40]. To increase inflammation, IL-17 induces mobilization, recruitment, and activation of different immune cells [40]. Interestingly, the finding of correlation between serum Galectin-3 levels and IL-17 production in patients with colorectal carcinoma has suggested that Galectin-3 may be one of the important modulators in the regulation of inflammatory conditions (**Figure 2**, [41]).

IL-17A (commonly referred to as IL-17) is the first discovered and best characterized member of the IL-17 family. Currently, six structurally related cytokines of IL-17 family have been identified (IL-17A to IL-17F) [42]. It is well documented that IL-17 plays protective role in infections, but here, we will review the multifunctional impacts of IL-17 on tumor biology.

IL-17 is mostly produced and secreted by Th17 lymphocytes, but it can be also produced by a broad spectrum of other cell populations [42]. Many studies describe the Th17-rich microenvironment in various types of tumor and that Th17 lymphocytes are endowed with a unique functional plasticity [40, 43]. Tumor cells, CAFs, and myeloid-derived suppressor cells (MDSCs) have been found to produce cytokine milieu that elicits recruitment and/or generation of Th17 lymphocytes [44, 45]. In addition, metabolic conditions present in the tumor milieu including indoleamine

2,3-dioxygenase (IDO) and hypoxia drive the differentiation of CD4 + T lymphocytes toward the Th17 lineage [46, 47]. Type 17 CD8 + T cytotoxic (Tc17) lymphocytes among tumor-infiltrating lymphocytes (TILs) were detected in nasopharyngeal [48] and gastric cancer [49]. Further, the main IL-17-producing cells in breast cancer are tumor-infiltrating γδT cells [50], and it seems that these TILs can promote the breast cancer progression [51]. NKT cells and group 3 innate lymphoid cells (ILC3s) represent other innate lymphocytes capable to produce IL-17 in the tumor microenvironment [52]. On the other hand, IL-17R is widely expressed in ECs, epithelial cells, fibroblasts, hematopoietic cells [53], and tumor cells [54], which implicates pleiotropic effects of IL-17 in the tumor microenvironment.

It seems that IL-17, as Roman god Janus, exerts two opposite faces in the tumor: "dark face" that drives tumor progression and "light face" responsible for the development of effective antitumor immunity. By *in vitro* and *in vivo* experiments, IL-17 signaling was shown to be "malevolent player" that promotes tumorigenesis and tumor progression, in many ways. In general, IL-17 exerts pro-tumor properties by direct influence on the tumor cells *via* triggering malignant transformation and tumor growth [55, 56] and/or indirectly by controlling chronic inflammatory and immunosuppressive tumor microenvironment, as well as angiogenesis [40, 57]. The IL-17/IL-17R axis upregulates phosphorylated ERK1/2 in breast cancer cells lines thereby promoting their proliferation, migration, and invasion [58]. Also, IL-17 can indirectly support the cell proliferation and tumor growth by shaping of tumor microenvironment through the production of chemokines and cytokines [59]. IL-17 was shown to be able to promote hepatocellular carcinoma invasion and migration by upregulation of matrix metalloproteases, MMP-2, and MMP-9, *via* NF-κB signaling [60]. IL-17 promotes STAT3 activity in both tumor and stromal cells, leading to upregulation of anti-apoptotic Bcl-2 and Bcl-XL in an IL-6-dependent manner [61]. This may reflect the fact that IL-17 present in the tumor microenvironment may be an important survival factor and reason for tumor chemoresistance. Accordingly, IL-17 promotes resistance of breast cancer cells to chemotherapeutic docetaxel *via* activation of ERK1/2 pathway [58]. Based on these findings, it can be speculated that IL-17 contributes to development of chemoresistance in variety tumor cells *via* activation of prosurvival and/or proliferative signaling. Recent evidence suggests that IL-17 links inflammation to tumor progression. Indeed, long-term IL-17 activity leads to pro-tumor microenvironment by inducing the secretion of inflammatory mediators and reshaping the phenotype of stromal cells [62]. Additionally, IL-17 stimulates the chemokine and VEGF expression that favor the recruitment of specific subsets of immune cells to the sites of inflammation and angiogenesis, respectively [63]. This IL-17-mediated maintenance of inflammatory environment results in the stimulation of tumor growth and metastasis *via* subsequent expression of anti-apoptotic molecules and increased tumor cell survival [64]. Ironically, Wang et al. [57] illustrated that IL-17, as pro-inflammatory cytokine, contributes to immune paralysis in the tumor microenvironment. Namely, IL-17 increases the expression of programmed death-ligand 1 (PD-L1) inhibitor on MSCs that shape the immunosuppressive environment and facilitate tumor progression. Further, chemokines (e.g., CXCL1 and CXCL5) stimulate the recruitment of MDSCs in IL-17-depandent manner to establish a proangiogenic and immunosuppressive tumor microenvironment [62]. Alongside its pro-tumorigenic functions, IL-17 may act as a tumor regressor. The protective role of IL-17 in tumor relies on its property to induce the vigorous immune responses to attain tumor regression. In fact, it has been demonstrated that effective antitumor immune response is mediated by Th17 lymphocytes and highly depends on IFN-γ [65]. Further, IL-17 enhances the CTLs-mediated immune response directed against hematopoietic tumors by induction of IL-6 and IL-12 production [40]. Therefore, IL-17 is multifunctional cytokine with divergent actions on tumor that are highly context-dependent. It seems that epigenetic and transcriptional modifications as well as certain cytokine milieu in the tumor microenvironment specific to each tumor type and stage may account for the functional plasticity of IL-17 making difficult to predict its role. Finally, IL-17 brings different net outcome in a complex disease such as tumor.

3. Galectin-3 as a tumor angiogenesis virtuoso

The critical events during angiogenic cascade such as activation, proliferation, and migration of ECs, as well as sprouting and tube formation, largely depend on Galectin-3 [66]. Initially, it has been observed that soluble Galectin-3 affects the migration of human umbilical vein endothelial cells (HUVECs) and capillary tube formation indicating its potential as chemoattractant for ECs [19]. This result has been confirmed by the increased tumor angiogenesis in the presence of Galectin-3 *in vivo*. The direct binding of Galectin-3 for endothelial cell surface appeared to be carbohydrate recognition-dependent event as it may be inhibited by disaccharide lactose and modified citrus pectin (MCP) [19, 67, 68].

Ever since, Galectin-3 has been widely recognized as powerful pro-angiogenic molecule acting through various receptors on the ECs, subsequently activating distinct signaling pathways involved in tumor angiogenesis (**Figure 2**). Interactions between Galectin-3 and different integrins expressed on ECs supposed to be critical in controlling endothelial cell migration and adhesion. Pericyte-derived neural/glial antigen 2 (NG2) proteoglycan, Galectin-3, and α3β1 integrin form the membrane complex that triggers intracellular signaling involved in endothelial cell motility [69]. The blocking antibodies specific for αVβ3, α5β1, and α2β1 integrins interfere with endothelial cell adhesion to Galectin-3-coated surface [70]. In addition to integrins, Galectin-3 on endothelial cell migration markedly depends on direct binding to the membrane highly glycosylated cell adhesion molecule CD146, also known as melanoma cell adhesion molecule [71]. CD146 has been recognized as VEGFR-2 co-receptor and a potential target for anti-angiogenic therapy in tumors [72]. The interaction between Galectin-3 and CD146 is also responsible for secretion of pro-metastatic cytokines by ECs indicating that this axis regulates distinct events during tumor progression [73]. Galectin-3 interacts with glycoprotein endoglin expressed predominantly by ECs as a component of TGF-β receptor complex [74]. Endoglin is abundantly expressed by proliferating ECs indicating an important role of TGF-β/endoglin signaling in tumor vasculature formation [75]. Therefore, thanks to its carbohydrate-binding capacity, Galectin-3 interacts with different molecules expressed by ECs in tumor microenvironment. Moreover, truncated Galectin-3, containing CRD domain, interacts more efficiently with ECs in comparison with full-length molecule [76, 77]. Apart from CRD domain, it seems that angiostimulatory effect of Galectin-3 also depends on its N-terminal tail [78]. Full-length Galectin-3, including its ability to oligomerize through N-terminal domain, appears to be necessary to affect migration of ECs and capillary tube formation [78]. Taken together, angiostimulatory effect of Galectin-3 on distinct events during angiogenesis has been mediated by different parts of the molecule in both carbohydrate dependent and independent manner [68].

Further investigation of the molecular mechanisms responsible for Galectin-3 pro-angiogenic actions in tumors documented its involvement in modulation of VEGF and basic fibroblast growth factor (bFGF) signaling pathways. Galectin-3 binds N-glycans of integrin $\alpha v\beta 3$ *via* CRD thus promoting its clustering and subsequent activation of focal adhesion kinase (FAK) in ECs [78]. FAK is a principal regulator of endothelial cell migration, proliferation, and survival, which participates in signal transduction triggered by integrins and growth factor receptors such as VEGFRs [79]. The expression of VEGFR-2, a major mediator of VEGF effects on ECs, is tightly regulated by FAK activation, its translocation to the nucleus, and subsequent regulation of VEGFR-2 gene transcription [79]. Given its carbohydrate-binding properties, Galectin-3 engages different N-glycosylated tyrosine kinase receptors including VEGFR-2 or FGF receptor-1 (FGFR-1) [80, 81]. It has been documented that Galectin-3 induces VEGFR-2 signaling during angiogenesis through modulation of expression and clustering of receptor on the ECs thus enabling its higher availability to VEGF [81]. However, the recent study has revealed that Galectin-3 amplifies the activation of VEGFR-2 and its downstream signaling only in the presence of VEGF [82]. Moreover, Galectin-3 is not necessary for VEGF-induced activation of VEGFR-2, nor it can activate the receptor in the absence of VEGF [82].

Galectin-3 has been described as a regulator of Jagged-1 (JAG1)/NOTCH1 signaling axis involved in tumor vasculature formation, in particular sprouting angiogenesis [83]. Under hypoxic condition, secreted Galectin-3 directly binds Notch ligand JAG1 in ECs thus activating pro-angiogenic JAG1/NOTCH1 signaling pathway. Galectin-3 prolongs the half-life of JAG1 over the Delta-like-4 (DLL4) thus affecting the balance between these molecules with opposite functions during angiogenic cascade [83, 84]. Interestingly, the proposed mechanism seems to be independent of VEGF/VEGFR signaling thus revealing novel potential targets in anti-angiogenic therapy.

In addition, Galectin-3 promotes the progression of hepatocellular carcinoma, including angiogenesis, through upregulation of β-catenin signaling [85]. Given its presence in different cellular compartments including nucleus, as well as its pleiotropic functions, Galectin-3 interferes with β-catenin pathway known to be active in various types of tumor. Galectin-3 activates PI3K/AKT signaling thus enhancing the phosphorylation and inactivation of key molecule of β-catenin degradation complex known as glycogen synthase kinase-3β (GSK-3β) [85, 86]. Subsequently, β-catenin accumulates in the nucleus and regulates the expression of genes involved in Galectin-3-mediated angiogenesis and epithelial-mesenchymal transition (EMT) [85].

Exosomes are vesicles secreted by living cells that participate in intercellular communication during essential processes such as proliferation, apoptosis, migration, and angiogenesis [87]. A highly glycosylated protein named lectin galactoside-binding soluble 3 binding protein (LGALS3BP), as a ligand for Galectin-3, has been previously recognized as a modulator of breast cancer angiogenesis that elevates VEGF expression via PI3K/AKT signaling pathway [88]. It has been shown recently that exosomes highly containing LGALS3BP affect endometrial cancer growth and angiogenesis [89]. The exosomes delivering LGALS3BP induce tumor cell proliferation and migration and HUVEC angiogenesis by triggering PI3K/AKT/VEGF signaling pathway [89].

The complex interplay between immunosuppression and angiogenesis is the integral part of tumor progression [29]. TAMs are the critical participants in tumor progression involved in the creation of immunosuppressive microenvironment thus enhancing metastasis and angiogenesis [90]. TAMs produce various pro-angiogenic molecules including growth factors (e.g., VEGF), chemokines, cytokines, as well as MMPs [90]. Galectin-3 promotes alternative activation of TAMs toward their pro-tumorigenic M2 phenotype (**Figure 2**, [29]). Increased angiogenesis in tumor is strongly associated with macrophage influx driven by elevated Galectin-3 expression [36]. Furthermore, Galectin-3 deficiency in both tumor tissue and stroma impairs angiogenesis *via* interfering with the responses of macrophages to the complex two-way VEGF and TGFβ-1 signaling pathways [91].

Collectively, thanks to its distinctive structure, Galectin-3 engages plenty of ligands both intracellularly and extracellularly, further interfering with various signaling pathways that regulate tumor angiogenesis. As a potential orchestrator of angiogenic cascade, Galectin-3 may be successfully targeted for anti-angiogenic tumor therapy.

4. Cytokine regulation of tumor angiogenesis: pro-angiogenic activity of IL-17

Apart from galectins, certain cytokine network within the tumor microenvironment contributes to angiogenesis mainly through sophisticated interplay between different cells and extracellular matrix components as well as stimulation of key pro-angiogenic mediator productions.

The data from human subjects have indicated the strong association between increased angiogenicity and high frequency of tumor-infiltrating Th17 lymphocytes [92, 93]. IL-17 overexpression has been associated with higher microvascular density (MVD) in tumors [92]. In general, IL-17 indirectly amplifies angiogenesis mostly by inducing VEGF upregulation, as well as another angiogenic factors by tumor cells and CAFs [94–96]. Also, IL-17 induces the recruitment of inflammatory cells with angiogenic phenotype (e.g., macrophages and neutrophils) and immunosuppressive cells to the tumor microenvironment, which contributes to different points of angiogenesis in many ways (**Figure 2**, [59, 97]). Even though the IL-17 overexpression has been detected in tumors, mechanisms of IL-17 that contribute to angiogenesis are still unclear. IL-17/IL-17RA axis promotes the activation of JAK-STAT3 signaling pathway resulting in phosphorylation and nuclear translocation of STAT3 [98]. STAT3 is important regulator of VEGF expression [96]. Furthermore, IL-17-mediated tumor angiogenesis involves the activation of STAT3/GIV (Gα-interacting vesicle-associated protein, Girdin) signaling pathway and subsequent upregulation of its downstream target VEGF [99]. Wu et al. [96] determined that IL-17 induces VEGF upregulation and neovascularization through STAT3-mediated signaling pathway in tumor cells that could be blocked by JSI-124, an inhibitor of phosphorylated STAT3. In addition, other mediators such as granulocyte colony-stimulating factor (G-CSF), EGF, FGF, PDGF, and IL-6 exhibit their pro-angiogenic functions *via* STAT3 signaling [61, 100]. IL-17 exerts synergistic effects with TNF-α by enhancing the secretion of potent angiogenic factors by stromal fibroblasts [94], which in turn triggers the angiogenic program in ECs and stimulates the new blood vessel development [95]. The inhibition of IL-17 suppresses VEGF expression in tumor tissue and decreases intratumoral MVD, which confirms important role of IL-17 in angiogenesis [101].

IL-17 stimulates the production of IL-8 [102]. IL-8 acts directly on ECs by promoting their proliferation, survival, and migration, as well as indirectly by increasing the recruitment of neutrophils that are important source of angiogenic factors in tumor microenvironment [103]. IL-17 activates ECs to produce pro-inflammatory chemokines and cytokines, including CXCL1, IL-8, and granulocyte macrophage-colony-stimulating factor (GM-CSF), thus promoting neutrophil recruitment and adhesion to ECs [98]. It is well known that neutrophils release plethora of molecules that promotes angiogenesis. In particular, neutrophil-derived MMP-9 is critical for catalyzing angiogenic switch in tumor cells and releasing of sequestered growth factors (e.g., VEGF), as well as remodeling of extracellular matrix (ECM) components during angiogenesis [104].

Accumulation of neutrophils has been associated with higher MVD and therefore more aggressive phenotype of gastric cancer [105]. IL-17 enhances the production of many angiogenic CXC chemokines including CXCL1, CXCL5, CXCL6, and CXCL8 (IL-8) [106, 107]. Among these, CXCL1 and CXCL5 are the important chemoattractants for neutrophils [108]. The listed chemokines also promote CXCR2-dependent angiogenesis by stimulating the migration and proliferation of ECs [107]. On the other hand, IL-17 facilitates recruitment and activation of MDSCs in tumor microenvironment [109]. Apart from immunosuppressive activity, MDSCs modulate angiogenesis *via* different mechanisms. Mostly, MDSCs stimulate angiogenesis by secreting numerous growth factors including VEGF, bFGF, and PDGF. They also remodel ECM components *via* MMPs production and reprogramming of other cells to tumor-promoting phenotype that are source of many angiogenesis activators [110].

Increased IL-17 and IL-23 mRNA expression has been associated with invasive gastric cancer [111]. We have shown that serum levels of IL-17 and IL-23 are significantly elevated in patients with colorectal carcinoma, but only IL-23 significantly correlated with overexpression of VEGF [112, 113]. It seems that IL-23 induces tumor-associated inflammation and angiogenesis thus promoting tumor growth [114]. IL-23-induced differentiation of Th17 lymphocytes suggests the possible indirect role of IL-23 in angiogenesis in IL-17-dependent manner (**Figure 2**).

There is evidence of tightly relationship between IL-17 and IL-33. Serum IL-33 has been associated with elevated IL-17 levels in patients with autoimmune hepatitis [115]. In addition, intestinal epithelial cells-derived IL-33 stimulates the recruitment of Th17 lymphocytes as the main cellular source of IL-17 in the small intestine [116]. Further, IL-6 can be critical trigger of IL-17 production, suggesting that the IL-33/IL-6/IL-17 axis plays a potential role in tumor biology [117]. It is well known that IL-33 is another pro-inflammatory cytokine with strong pro-angiogenic capacity (**Figure 2**). Similar to IL-17, IL-33 promotes the production of different pro-angiogenic factors, including VEGF and IL-8 [118]. It appears that IL-33 increases endothelial cell proliferation and vascular permeability [119]. Milosavljevic et al. [120] have found significantly higher expression of IL-33, IL-33 receptor, and VEGF in breast cancer. IL-33 and IL-33R expression correlated with VEGF expression in tumor tissue. VEGF expression positively correlated with MVD implicating that IL-33/IL-33R pathway is involved in breast cancer growth [120]. Further, tumor-derived IL-33 induces the recruitment of CD11b + Gr1+ and CD11b + F4/80+ myeloid cells to the tumor microenvironment further contributing to angiogenesis *via* different mechanisms [121]. IL-33/ST2 axis rapidly increased NO production through TRAF6-mediated activation of PI3K, AKT, and NO synthase in the ECs [119]. Also, AKT signaling in the ECs is transiently regulated by angiogenic factors such as VEGF and angiopoietin-1 [122]. Taken together, the better understanding of cytokine-regulated angiogenesis, notably by IL-17, is of great importance for the rational development of new tumor therapeutic strategies.

5. Galectin-3 and IL-17 in anti-angiogenic tumor therapy

Angiogenesis is complex and dynamic process in which more actors take part. To date, several anti-angiogenic agents, mainly acting *via* targeting VEGF and its receptor, have been in clinical use. It seems that the blockade of pro-angiogenic Galectin-3 and IL-17 might be the potential strategy to open opportunities for additional tumor immunotherapy, in particular in tumors that overexpress Galectin-3 and IL-17. It has been shown that IL-17 signaling pathways, notably, IL-17-mediated paracrine network in the tumor microenvironment, mediate tumor refractoriness to the anti-angiogenic effects of VEGF blockade [123, 124]. IL-17 induces expression of numerous cytokine, most notably, G-CSF that is essential for the development and recruitment of CD11b + Gr1+ MDSCs [97, 124] to the tumor microenvironment in which these "angiocompetent cells" probably take part in both VEGF-dependent and VEGF-independent angiogenesis [125]. Taken together, these data suggest that the inhibition of IL-17 signaling may render tumor sensitive to VEGF-targeting therapy and/or reduce the VEGF-independent tumor angiogenesis.

MCP is specifically inhibitor of Galectin-3, which significant decreases the MVD, suggesting that targeting Galectin-3 may open novel perspectives to interfere with tumor angiogenesis [67]. On the other hand, anti-angiogenic treatments have therapeutic limitations including varying degrees of response and resistance due to VEGF-independent mechanisms. Thus, VEGF blockade creates hypoxic conditions in the tumor, which in turn causes increased invasion and poorer survival by inducting of HIF-1α-dependent c-Met overexpression [126]. In hypoxic areas, tumor cells also survive oxygen-depleted environment by upregulating Galectin-3 expression, which may in turn increase tumor aggressiveness [127]. The simultaneous blockade of VEGF and Galectin-3 could be providing a more potent antitumor effect, which is mediated by, among others, anti-angiogenic mechanisms.

Finally, due to the fact that multiple actors are involved in tumor angiogenesis, Galectin-3 and IL-17 targeting is likely to improve the efficacy of current anti-angiogenic tumor therapy.

Acknowledgements

This work was supported by a grant from the Ministry of Education, Science and Technological Development, Serbia (ON175069 and ON175071), a bilateral project with People's Republic of China (06/2018) and by the Faculty of Medical Sciences of the University of Kragujevac, Serbia (JP16/19).

Author details

Gordana D. Radosavljevic*, Jelena Pantic, Bojana Simovic Markovic and Nebojsa Arsenijevic
Faculty of Medical Sciences, Center for Molecular Medicine and Stem Cell Research, University of Kragujevac, Kragujevac, Serbia

*Address all correspondence to: perun.gr@gmail.com

References

[1] Folkman J. Tumor angiogenesis: Therapeutic implications. The New England Journal of Medicine. 1971;**285**:1182-1186. DOI: 10.1056/NEJM197111182852108

[2] Nejad AE, Najafgholian S, Rostami A, Sistani A, Shojaeifar S, Esparvarinha M, et al. The role of hypoxia in the tumor microenvironment and development of cancer stem cell: A novel approach to developing treatment. Cancer Cell International. 2021;**21**:62. DOI: 10.1186/s12935-020-01719-5

[3] Lee SH, Jeong D, Han Y-S, Baek MJ. Pivotal role of vascular endothelial growth factor pathway in tumor angiogenesis. Annals of Surgical Treatment and Research. 2015l;**89**:1-8. DOI: 10.4174/astr.2015.89.1.1

[4] Nishida N, Yano H, Nishida T, Kamura T, Kojiro M. Angiogenesis in Cancer. Vascular Health and Risk Management. 2006;**2**:213-219. DOI: 10.2147/vhrm.2006.2.3.213

[5] Shibuya M, Claesson-Welsh L. Signal transduction by VEGF receptors in regulation of angiogenesis and lymphangiogenesis. Experimental Cell Research. 2006;**3125**:549-560. DOI: 10.1016/j.yexcr.2005.11.012

[6] Gee E, Milkiewicz M, Haas TL. p38 MAPK is activated by vascular endothelial growth factor receptor 2 and is essential for shear stress-induced angiogenesis. Journal of Cellular Physiology. 2010;**222**:120-126. DOI: 10.1002/jcp.21924

[7] Yang G-L, Li L-Y. Counterbalance: Modulation of VEGF/VEGFR activities by TNFSF15. Signal Transduction and Targeted Therapy. 2018;**3**:21. DOI: 10.1038/s41392-018-0023-8

[8] Dvorak HF, Brown LF, Detmar M, Dvorak AM. Vascular permeability factor/vascular endothelial growth factor, microvascular hyperpermeability, and angiogenesis. The American Journal of Pathology. 1995;**146**:1029-1039

[9] Meadows KN, Bryant P, Pumiglia K. Vascular endothelial growth factor induction of the angiogenic phenotype requires Ras activation. The Journal of Biological Chemistry. 2001;**276**:49289-49298. DOI: 10.1074/jbc.M108069200

[10] Gerber HP, Dixit V, Ferrara N. Vascular endothelial growth factor induces expression of the antiapoptotic proteins Bcl-2 and A1 in vascular endothelial cells. Journal of Biological Chemistry. 1998;**273**:13313-13316. DOI: 10.1074/jbc.273.21.13313

[11] Rafii S, Lyden D, Benezra R, Hattori K, Heissig B. Vascular and haematopoietic stem cells: Novel targets for anti-angiogenesis therapy? Nature Reviews. Cancer. 2002;**2**:826-835. DOI: 10.1038/nrc925

[12] Jiang BH, Liu LZ. PI3K/PTEN signaling in angiogenesis and tumorigenesis. Advances in Cancer Research. 2009;**102**:19-65. DOI: 10.1016/S0065-230X(09)02002-8

[13] Jiang X, Wang J, Deng X, Xiong F, Zhang S, Gong Z, et al. The role of microenvironment in tumor angiogenesis. Journal of Experimental & Clinical Cancer Research. 2020;**39**:204. DOI: 10.1186/s13046-020-01709-5

[14] Martin JD, Seano G, Jain RK. Normalizing function of tumor vessels: Progress, opportunities, and challenges. Annual Review of Physiology.

2019;**81**:505-534. DOI: 10.1146/annurev-physiol-020518-114700

[15] Wei F, Wang D, Wei J, Tang N, Tang L, Xiong F, et al. Metabolic crosstalk in the tumor microenvironment regulates antitumor immunosuppression and immunotherapy resisitance. Cellular and Molecular Life Sciences. 2020;**8**:284. DOI: 10.1007/s00018-020-03581-0

[16] Radosavljevic G, Volarevic V, Jovanovic I, Milovanovic M, Pejnovic N, Arsenijevic N, et al. The roles of Galectin-3 in autoimmunity and tumor progression. Immunologic Research. 2012;**52**:100-110. DOI: 10.1007/s12026-012-8286-6

[17] Radosavljevic GD, Pantic J, Jovanovic I, Lukic ML, Arsenijevic N. The two faces of Galectin-3: Roles in various pathological conditions. Serbian Journal of Experimental and Clinical Research. 2016;**17**:187-198. DOI: 10.1515/SJECR-2016-0011

[18] Caponc E, Iacobelli S, Sala G. Role of galectin 3 binding protein in cancer progression: A potential novel therapeutic target. Journal of Translational Medicine. 2021;**19**:405. DOI: 10.1186/s12967-021-03085-w

[19] Nangia Makker P, Honjo Y, Sarvis R, Akahani S, Hogan V, Pienta KJ, et al. Galectin 3 induces endothelial cell morphogenesis and angiogenesis. The American Journal of Pathology. 2000;**156**:899-909. DOI: 10.1016/S0002-9440(10)64959-0

[20] Henderson NC, Mackinnon AC, Farnworth SL, Poirier F, Russo FP, Iredale JP, et al. Galectin 3 regulates myofibroblast activation and hepatic fibrosis. Proceedings of the National Academy of Sciences of the United States of America. 2006;**103**:5060-5065. DOI: 10.1073/pnas.0511167103

[21] Sioud M, Mobergslien A, Boudabous A, Fløisand Y. Evidence for the involvement of galectin 3 in mesenchymal stem cell suppression of allogeneic T cell proliferation. Scandinavian Journal of Immunology. 2010;**71**:267-274. DOI: 10.1111/j.1365-3083.2010.02378.x

[22] Furuhata S, Ando K, Oki M, Aoki K, Ohnishi S, Aoyagi K, et al. Gene expression profiles of endothelial progenitor cells by oligonucleotide microarray analysis. Molecular and Cellular Biochemistry. 2007;**298**:125-138. DOI: 10.1007/s11010-006-9359-4

[23] Glinskii OV, Turk JR, Pienta KJ, Huxley VH, Glinsky VV. Evidence of porcine and human endothelium activation by cancer-associated carbohydrates expressed on glycoproteins and tumour cells. The Journal of Physiology. 2004;**554**:89-99. DOI: 10.1113/jphysiol.2003.054783

[24] Gil CD, La M, Perretti M, Oliani SM. Interaction of human neutrophils with endothelial cells regulates the expression of endogenous proteins annexin 1, galectin-1 and galectin-3. Cell Biology International. 2006;**30**:338-344. DOI: 10.1016/j.cellbi.2005.12.010

[25] Rao SP, Wang Z, Zuberi RI, Sikora L, Bahaie NS, Zuraw BL, et al. Galectin-3 functions as an adhesion molecule to support eosinophil rolling and adhesion under conditions of flow. Journal of Immunology. 2007;**179**:7800-7807. DOI: 10.4049/jimmunol.179.11

[26] Annese T, Tamma R, Ruggieri S, Ribatti D. Erythropoietin in tumor angiogenesis. Experimental Cell Research. 2019;**374**:266-273. DOI: 10.1016/j.yexcr.2018.12.013

[27] Ruvolo PP. Galectin 3 as a guardian of the tumor microenvironment.

Biochimica et Biophysica Acta. 2016;**1863**:427-437. DOI: 10.1016/j.bbamcr.2015.08.008

[28] Ahmed H, AlSadek DMM. Galectin-3 as a potential target to prevent Cancer metastasis. Clinical Medicine Insights: Oncology. 2015;**9**:113-121. DOI: 10.4137/CMO.S29462

[29] Farhad M, Rolig AS, Redmonda WL. The role of Galectin-3 in modulating tumor growth and immunosuppression within the tumor microenvironment. OncoImmunology. 2018;**7**:e1434467. DOI: 10.1080/2162402X.2018.1434467

[30] Wang L, Li Y-S, Yu L-G, Zhang X-K, Zhao L, Gong F-L, et al. Galectin-3 expression and secretion by tumor-associated macrophages in hypoxia promotes breast cancer progression. Biochemical Pharmacology. 2020;**178**:114113. DOI: 10.1016/j.bcp.2020.114113

[31] Çakır Y, Talu CK, Mermut Ö, Trabulus DC, Arslan E. The expression of Galectin-3 in tumor and Cancer-associated fibroblasts in invasive micropapillary breast carcinomas: Relationship with Clinicopathologic parameters. European Journal Of Breast Health. 2021;**17**:341-351. DOI: 10.4274/ejbh.galenos.2021.2021-2-8

[32] Escrevente C, Grammel N, Kandzia S, Zeiser J, Tranfield EM, Conradt HS, et al. Sialoglycoproteins and N-glycans from secreted exosomes of ovarian carcinoma cells. PLoS One. 2013;**8**:e78631. DOI: 10.1371/journal.pone.0078631

[33] Dange MC, Srinivasan N, More SK, Bane SM, Upadhya A, Ingle AD, et al. Galectin-3 expressed on different lung compartments promotes organ specific metastasis by facilitating arrest, extravasation and organ colonization via high affinity ligands on melanoma cells. Clinical & Experimental Metastasis. 2014;**31**:661-673. DOI: 10.1007/s10585-014-9657-2

[34] Radosavljevic G, Jovanovic I, Majstorovic M, Mitrovic M, Juranic Lisnic V, Arsenijevic N, et al. Deletion of Galectin-3 in the host attenuates metastasis of murine melanoma by modulating tumor adhesion and NK cell activity. Clinical & Experimental Metastasis. 2011;**28**:451-462. DOI: 10.1007/s10585-011-9383-y

[35] Aguilar-Cazares D, Chavez-Dominguez R, Carlos-Reyes A, Lopez-Camarillo C, Hernadez de la CruzON,Lopez-GonzalezJS.Contribution of angiogenesis to inflammation and Cancer. Frontiers in Oncology. 2019;**9**:1399. DOI: 10.3389/fonc.2019.01399

[36] Jia W, Kidoya H, Yamakawa D, Naito H, Takakura N. Galectin-3 accelerates M2 macrophage infiltration and angiogenesis in tumors. The American Journal of Pathology. 2013;**182**:1821-1831. DOI: 10.1016/j.ajpath.2013.01.017

[37] Chen C, Duckworth CA, Zhao Q, Pritchard DM, Rhodes JM, Yu L-G. Increased circulation of galectin-3 in cancer induces secretion of metastasis-promoting cytokines from blood vascular endothelium. Clinical Cancer Research. 2013;**19**:1693-1704. DOI: 10.1158/1078-0432.CCR-12-2940

[38] Goldberg JE, Schwertfeger KL. Proinflammatory cytokines in breast cancer: Mechanisms of action and potential targets for therapeutics. Current Drug Targets. 2010;**11**:1133-1146. DOI: 10.2174/138945010792006799

[39] Landskron G, De la Fuente M, Thuwajit P, Thuwajit C, Hermoso MA. Chronic inflammation and cytokines

in the tumor microenvironment. Journal of Immunology Research. 2014;**2014**:149185. DOI: 10.1155/2014/149185

[40] Murugaiyan G, Saha B. Protumor vs antitumor functions of IL-17. Journal of Immunology. 2009;**183**:4169-4175. DOI: 10.4049/jimmunol.0901017

[41] Shimura T, Shibata M, Gonda K, Nakajima T, Chida S, Noda M, et al. Association between circulating galectin-3 levels and the immunological, inflammatory and nutritional parameters in patients with colorectal cancer. Biomedical Reports. 2016;**5**:203-207. DOI: 10.3892/br.2016.696

[42] Yun G, Huang M, Yao Y-M. Biology of Interleukin-17 and its pathophysiological significance in Sepsis. Frontiers in Immunology. 2020;**11**:1558. DOI: 10.3389/fimmu.2020.01558

[43] Du J-W, Xu K-Y, Fang L-Y, Qi X-L. Interleukin-17, produced by lymphocytes, promotes tumor growth and angiogenesis in a mouse model of breast cancer. Molecular Medicine Reports. 2012;**6**:1099-1102. DOI: 10.3892/mmr.2012.1036

[44] Su X, Ye J, Hsueh EC, Zhang Y, Hoft DF, Peng G. Tumor microenvironments direct the recruitment and expansion of human Th17 cells. Journal of Immunology. 2010;**184**:1630-1641. DOI: 10.4049/jimmunol.0902813

[45] Chen C, Gao F-H. Th17 cells paradoxical roles in melanoma and potential application in immunotherapy. Frontiers in Immunology. 2019;**10**:187. DOI: 10.3389/fimmu.2019.00187

[46] Dang EV, Barbi J, Yang H-Y, Jinasena D, Yu H, Zheng Y, et al. Control of T(H)17/T(reg) balance by hypoxia-inducible factor 1. Cell. 2011;**146**:772-784. DOI: 10.1016/j.cell.2011.07.033

[47] Sharma MD, Hou D-Y, Liu Y, Koni PA, Metz R, Chandler P, et al. Indoleamine 2,3-dioxygenase controls conversion of Foxp3+ Tregs to TH17-like cells in tumor-draining lymph nodes. Blood. 2009;**113**:6102-6111. DOI: 10.1182/blood-2008-12-1953

[48] Li J, Huang Z-F, Xiong G, Mo H-Y, Qiu F, Mai H-Q, et al. Distribution, characterization, and induction of CD8+ regulatory T cells and IL-17-producing CD8+ T cells in nasopharyngeal carcinoma. Journal of Translational Medicine. 2011;**9**:189. DOI: 10.1186/1479-5876-9-189

[49] Zhuang Y, Peng L-S, Zhao Y-L, Shi Y, Mao X-H, Chen W, et al. CD8(+) T cells that produce interleukin-17 regulate myeloid-derived suppressor cells and are associated with survival time of patients with gastric cancer. Gastroenterology. 2012;**143**:951-62.e8. DOI: 10.1053/j.gastro.2012.06.010

[50] Meng S, Li L, Zhou M, Jiang W, Niu H, Yang K. Distribution and prognostic value of tumor-infiltrating T cells in breast cancer. Molecular Medicine Reports. 2018;**18**:4247-4258. DOI: 10.3892/mmr.2018.9460

[51] Patin EC, Soulard D, Fleury S, Hassane M, Dombrowicz D, Faveeuw C, et al. Type I IFN receptor Signaling controls IL7-dependent accumulation and activity of Protumoral IL17A-producing γδT cells in breast Cancer. Cancer Research. 2018;**78**:195-204. DOI: 10.1158/0008-5472.CAN-17-1416

[52] Kuen D-S, Kim B-S, Chung Y. IL-17-producing cells in tumor immunity: Friends or foes? Immune Network. 2020;**20**:e6. DOI: 10.4110/in.2020.20.e6

[53] Chang SH, Dong C. Signaling of interleukin-17 family cytokines in immunity and inflammation. Cellular Signalling. 2011;**23**:1069-1075. DOI: 10.1016/j.cellsig.2010.11.022

[54] Jiang Y-X, Li P-A, Yang S-W, Hao Y-X, Yu P-W. Increased chemokine receptor IL-17RA expression is associated with poor survival in gastric cancer patients. International Journal of Clinical and Experimental Pathology. 2015;**8**:7002-7008

[55] Kim G, Khanal P, Lim SC, Yun HJ, Ahn SG, Ki SH, et al. Interleukin-17 induces AP-1 activity and cellular transformation via upregulation of tumor progression locus 2 activity. Carcinogenesis. 2013;**34**:341-350. DOI: 10.1093/carcin/bgs342

[56] Nam JS, Terabe M, Kang MJ, Chae H, Voong N, Yang YA, et al. Transforming growth factor β subverts the immune system into directly promoting tumor growth through interleukin-17. Cancer Research. 2008;**68**:3915-3923. DOI: 10.1158/0008-5472.CAN-08-0206

[57] Wang S, Wang G, Zhang L, Li F, Liu K, Wang Y, et al. Interleukin 17 promotes nitric oxide dependent expression of PD L1 in mesenchymal stem cells. Cell & Bioscience. 2020;**10**:73. DOI: 10.1186/s13578-020-00431-1

[58] Cochaud S, Giustiniani J, Thomas C, Laprevotte E, Garbar C, Savoye A-M, et al. IL-17A is produced by breast cancer TILs and promotes chemoresistance and proliferation through ERK1/2. Scientific Reports. 2013;**3**:3456. DOI: 10.1038/srep03456

[59] Vitiello GA, Miller G. Targeting the interleukin-17 immune axis for cancer immunotherapy. The Journal of Experimental Medicine. 2020;**217**:e20190456. DOI: 10.1084/jem.20190456

[60] Li J, Lau GK, Chen L, Dong SS, Lan HY, Huang XR, et al. Interleukin 17A promotes hepatocellular carcinoma metastasis via NF-kB induced matrix metalloproteinases 2 and 9 expression. PLoS One. 2011;**6**:e21816. DOI: 10.1371/journal.pone.0021816

[61] Wang L, Yi T, Kortylewski M, Pardoll DM, Zeng D, Yu H. IL-17 can promote tumor growth through an IL-6-Stat3 signaling pathway. The Journal of Experimental Medicine. 2009;**206**:1457-1464. DOI: 10.1084/jem.20090207

[62] Zhao J, Chen X, Herjan T, Li X. The role of interleukin-17 in tumor development and progression. The Journal of Experimental Medicine. 2020;**217**:e20190297. DOI: 10.1084/jem.20190297

[63] Welte T, Zhang XH-F. Interleukin-17 could promote breast Cancer progression at several stages of the disease. Mediators of Inflammation. 2015;**2015**:804347. DOI: 10.1155/2015/804347

[64] Yang B, Kang H, Fung A, Zhao H, Wang T, Ma D. The role of interleukin 17 in tumour proliferation, angiogenesis, and metastasis. Mediators of Inflammation. 2014;**2014**:623759. DOI: 10.1155/2014/623759

[65] Muranski P, Boni A, Antony PA, Cassard L, Irvine KR, Kaiser A, et al. Tumor-specific Th17-polarized cells eradicate large established melanoma. Blood. 2008;**112**:362-373. DOI: 10.1182/blood-2007-11-120998

[66] Thijssen VL. Galectins in endothelial cell biology and angiogenesis: The basics. Biomolecules. 2021;**11**:1386. DOI: 10.3390/biom11091386

[67] Nangia-Makker P, Hogan V, Honjo Y, Baccarini S, Tait L, Bresalier R, et al. Inhibition of human cancer cell

growth and metastasis in nude mice by oral intake of modified citrus pectin. Journal of the National Cancer Institute. 2002;**94**:1854-1862. DOI: 10.1093/jnci/94.24.1854

[68] Funasaka T, Raz A, Nangia-Makker P. Galectin-3 in angiogenesis and metastasis. Glycobiology. 2014;**24**:886-891. DOI: 10.1093/glycob/cwu086

[69] Fukushi J, Makagiansar IT, Stallcup WB. NG2 proteoglycan promotes endothelial cell motility and angiogenesis via engagement of Galectin-3 and α3β1 integrin. Molecular Biology of the Cell. 2004;**15**:3580-3590. DOI: 10.1091/mbc.e04-03-0236

[70] Sedlář A, Trávníčková M, Bojarová P, Vlachová M, Slámová K, Křen V, et al. Interaction between Galectin-3 and Integrins mediates cell-matrix adhesion in endothelial cells and mesenchymal stem cells. International Journal of Molecular Sciences. 2021;**22**:5144. DOI: 10.3390/ijms22105144

[71] Zhang Z, Zheng Y, Wang H, Zhou Y, Tai G. CD146 interacts with galectin-3 to mediate endothelial cell migration. FEBS Letters. 2018;**592**:1817-1828. DOI: 10.1002/1873-3468.13083

[72] Jiang T, Zhuang J, Duan H, Luo Y, Zeng Q, Fan K, et al. CD146 is a coreceptor for VEGFR-2 in tumor angiogenesis. Blood. 2012;**120**:2330-2339. DOI: 10.1182/blood-2012-01-406108

[73] Colomb F, Wang W, Simpson D, Zafar M, Beynon R, Rhodes JM, et al. Galectin-3 interacts with the cell-surface glycoprotein CD146 (MCAM, MUC18) and induces secretion of metastasis-promoting cytokines from vascular endothelial cells. Journal of Biological Chemistry. 2017;**292**:8381-8389. DOI: 10.1074/jbc.M117.783431

[74] Gallardo-Vara E, Ruiz-Llorente L, Casado-Vela J, Ruiz-Rodríguez MJ, López-Andrés N, Pattnaik AK, et al. Endoglin protein Interactome profiling identifies TRIM21 and Galectin-3 as new binding partners. Cell. 2019;**8**:1082. DOI: 10.3390/cells8091082

[75] Bernabeu C, Lopez-Novoa JM, Quintanilla M. The emerging role of TGF-beta superfamily coreceptors in cancer. Biochimica et Biophysica Acta. 2009;**1792**:954-973. DOI: 10.1016/j.bbadis.2009.07.003

[76] Nangia-Makker P, Raz T, Tait L, Hogan V, Fridman R, Raz A. Galectin-3 cleavage: A novel surrogate marker for matrix metalloproteinase activity in growing breast cancers. Cancer Research. 2007;**67**:11760-11768. DOI: 10.1158/0008-5472.CAN-07-323

[77] Nangia-Makker P, Wang Y, Raz T, Tait L, Balan V, Hogan V, et al. Cleavage of galectin-3 by matrix metalloproteases induces angiogenesis in breast cancer. International Journal of Cancer. 2010;**127**:2530-2541. DOI: 10.1002/ijc.25254

[78] Markowska AI, Liu FT, Panjwani N. Galectin-3 is an important mediator of VEGF- and bFGF-mediated angiogenic response. The Journal of Experimental Medicine. 2010;**207**:1981-1993. DOI: 10.1084/jem.20090121

[79] Sun S, Wu HJ, Guan JL. Nuclear FAK and its kinase activity regulate VEGFR2 transcription in angiogenesis of adult mice. Scientific Reports. 2018;**8**:2550. DOI: 10.1038/s41598-018-20930-z

[80] Markowska AI, Jefferies KC, Panjwani N. Galectin-3 protein modulates cell surface expression and activation of vascular endothelial growth factor receptor 2 in human endothelial cells. The Journal of Biological

Chemistry. 2011;**286**:29913-29921. DOI: 10.1074/jbc.M111.226423

[81] Kucińska M, Porębska N, Lampart A, Latko M, Knapik A, Zakrzewska M, et al. Differential regulation of fibroblast growth factor receptor 1 trafficking and function by extracellular galectins. Cell Communication and Signaling: CCS. 2019;**17**:65. DOI: 10.1186/s12964-019-0371-1

[82] Cano I, Hu Z, AbuSamra DB, Saint-Geniez M, Ng YSE, Argüeso P, et al. Galectin-3 enhances vascular endothelial growth factor-a receptor 2 activity in the presence of vascular endothelial growth factor. Frontiers in Cell and Development Biology. 2021;**9**:734346. DOI: 10.3389/fcell.2021.734346

[83] Dos Santos SN, Sheldon H, Pereira JX, Paluch C, Bridges EM, El-Cheikh MC, et al. Galectin-3 acts as an angiogenic switch to induce tumor angiogenesis via Jagged-1/notch activation. Oncotarget. 2017;**8**:49484-49501. DOI: 10.18632/oncotarget.17718

[84] Benedito R, Roca C, Sorensen I, Adams S, Gossler A, Fruttiger M, et al. The notch ligands Dll4 and Jagged1 have opposing effects on angiogenesis. Cell. 2009;**137**:1124-1135. DOI: 10.1016/j.cell.2009.03.025

[85] Song M, Pan Q, Yang J, He J, Zeng J, Cheng S, et al. Galectin-3 favours tumour metastasis via the activation of β-catenin signalling in hepatocellular carcinoma. British Journal of Cancer. 2020;**123**:1521-1534. DOI: 10.1038/s41416-020-1022-4

[86] Song S, Mazurek N, Liu C, Sun Y, Ding QQ, Liu K, et al. Galectin-3 mediates nuclear beta-catenin accumulation and Wnt signaling in human colon cancer cells by regulation of glycogen synthase kinase-3beta activity. Cancer Research. 2009;**69**:1343-1349. DOI: 10.1158/0008-5472.CAN-08-4153

[87] Gurung S, Perocheau D, Touramanidou L, Baruteau J. The exosome journey: From biogenesis to uptake and intracellular signaling. Cell Communication and Signaling: CCS. 2021;**19**:47. DOI: 10.1186/s12964-021-00730-1

[88] Piccolo E, Tinari N, Semeraro D, Traini S, Fichera I, Cumashi A, et al. LGALS3BP, lectin galactoside-binding soluble 3 binding protein, induces vascular endothelial growth factor in human breast cancer cells and promotes angiogenesis. Journal of Molecular Medicine (Berlin, Germany). 2013;**91**:83-94. DOI: 10.1007/s00109-012-0936-6

[89] Song Y, Wang M, Tong H, Tan Y, Hu X, Wang K, et al. Plasma exosomes from endometrial cancer patients contain LGALS3BP to promote endometrial cancer progression. Oncogene. 2021;**40**:633-646. DOI: 10.1038/s41388-020-01555-x

[90] Fu LQ, Du WL, Cai MH, Yao JY, Zhao YY, Mou XZ. The roles of tumor-associated macrophages in tumor angiogenesis and metastasis. Cellular Immunology. 2020;**353**:104119. DOI: 10.1016/j.cellimm.2020.104119

[91] Machado CM, Andrade LN, Teixeira VR, Costa FF, Melo CM, dos Santos SN, et al. Galectin-3 disruption impaired tumoral angiogenesis by reducing VEGF secretion from TGFb1-induced macrophages. Cancer Medicine. 2014;**3**:201-214. DOI: 10.1002/cam4.173

[92] Liu J, Duan Y, Cheng X, Chen X, Xie W, Long H, et al. IL-17 is associated with poor prognosis and promotes angiogenesis via stimulating VEGF production of cancer cells in colorectal carcinoma. Biochemical and

Biophysical Research Communications. 2011;**407**:348-354. DOI: 10.1016/j.bbrc.2011.03.021

[93] Zhang JP, Yan J, Xu J, Pang XH, Chen MS, Li L, et al. Increased intratumoral IL-17-producing cells correlate with poor survival in hepatocellular carcinoma patients. Journal of Hepatology. 2009;**50**:980-989. DOI: 10.1016/j.jhep.2008.12.033

[94] Numasaki M, Lotze MT, Sasaki H. Interleukin-17 augments tumor necrosis factor-alpha-induced elaboration of proangiogenic factors from fibroblasts. Immunology Letters. 2004;**93**:39-43. DOI: 10.1016/j.imlet.2004.01.014

[95] Takahashi H, Numasaki M, Lotze MT, Sasaki H. Interleukin-17 enhances bFGF-, HGF- and VEGF-induced growth of vascular endothelial cells. Immunology Letters. 2005;**98**:189-193. DOI: 10.1016/j.imlet.2004.11.012

[96] Wu X, Yang T, Liu X, Nian Guo J, Xie T, Ding Y, et al. IL-17 promotes tumor angiogenesis through Stat3 pathway mediated upregulation of VEGF in gastric cancer. Tumour Biology. 2016;**37**:5493-5501. DOI: 10.1007/s13277-015-4372-4

[97] He D, Li H, Yusuf N, Elmets CA, Li J, Mountz JD, et al. IL-17 promotes tumor development through the induction of tumor promoting microenvironments at tumor sites and myeloid-derived suppressor cells. Journal of Immunology. 2010;**184**:2281-2288. DOI: 10.4049/jimmunol.0902574

[98] Yuan S, Zhang S, Zhuang Y, Zhang H, Bai J, Hou Q. Interleukin-17 stimulates STAT3-mediated endothelial cell activation for neutrophil recruitment. Cellular Physiology and Biochemistry. 2015;**36**(6):2340-2356. DOI: 10.1159/000430197

[99] Pan B, Shen J, Cao J, Zhou Y, Shang L, Jin S, et al. Interleukin-17 promotes angiogenesis by stimulating VEGF production of cancer cells via the STAT3/GIV signaling pathway in non-small-cell lung cancer. Scientific Reports. 2020;**10**:8808. DOI: 10.1038/s41598-020-65650-5

[100] Levy DE, Darnell JE Jr. Stats: Transcriptional control and biological impact. Nature Reviews. Molecular Cell Biology. 2002;**3**:651-662. DOI: 10.1038/nrm909

[101] Hayata K, Iwahashi M, Ojima T, Katsuda M, Iida T, Nakamori M, et al. Inhibition of IL-17A in tumor microenvironment augments cytotoxicity of tumor-infiltrating lymphocytes in tumor-bearing mice. PLoS One. 2013;**8**:e53131. DOI: 10.1371/journal.pone.0053131

[102] Kehlen A, Thiele K, Riemann D, Rainov N, Langner J. Interleukin-17 stimulates the expression of IkappaB alpha mRNA and the secretion of IL-6 and IL-8 in glioblastoma cell lines. Journal of Neuroimmunology. 1999;**101**:1-6. DOI: 10.1016/s0165-5728(99)00111-3

[103] Waugh DJJ, Wilson C. The interleukin-8 pathway in cancer. Clinical Cancer Research. 2008;**14**:6735-6741. DOI: 10.1158/1078-0432.CCR-07-4843

[104] Ardi VC, Kupriyanova TA, Deryugina EI, Quigley JP. Human neutrophils uniquely release TIMP-free MMP-9 to provide a potent catalytic stimulator of angiogenesis. Proceedings of the National Academy of Sciences of the United States of America. 2007;**104**:20262-20267. DOI: 10.1073/pnas.0706438104

[105] Su Z, Sun Y, Zhu H, Liu Y, Lin X, Shen H, et al. Th17 cell expansion in

gastric cancer may contribute to cancer development and metastasis. Immunologic Research. 2014;**58**:118-124. DOI: 10.1007/s12026-013-8483-y

[106] Numasaki M, Watanabe M, Suzuki T, Takahashi H, Nakamura A, McAllister F, et al. IL-17 enhances the net angiogenic activity and in vivo growth of human non-small cell lung cancer in SCID mice through promoting CXCR-2-dependent angiogenesis. Journal of Immunology. 2005;**175**:6177-6189. DOI: 10.4049/jimmunol.175.9.6177

[107] Keeley EC, Mehrad B, Strieter RM. Chemokines as mediators of tumor angiogenesis and neovascularization. Experimental Cell Research. 2011;**317**:685-690. DOI: 10.1016/j.yexcr.2010.10.020

[108] Fridlender ZG, Sun J, Kim S, Kapoor V, Cheng G, Ling L, et al. Polarization of tumor-associated neutrophil phenotype by TGF-beta: "N1" versus "N2" TAN. Cancer Cell. 2009;**16**:183-194. DOI: 10.1016/j.ccr.2009.06.017

[109] Parker KH, Beury DW, Ostrand-Rosenberg S. Myeloid-derived suppressor cells: Critical cells driving immune suppression in the tumor microenvironment. Advances in Cancer Research. 2015;**128**:95-139. DOI: 10.1016/bs.acr.2015.04.002

[110] Vetsika E-K, Koukos A, Kotsakis A. Myeloid-derived suppressor cells: Major figures that shape the immunosuppressive and Angiogenic network in Cancer. Cell. 2019;**8**:1647. DOI: 10.3390/cells8121647

[111] Iida T, Iwahashi M, Katsuda M, Ishida K, Nakamori M, Nakamura M, et al. Tumor-infiltrating CD4+ Th17 cells produce IL-17 in tumor microenvironment and promote tumor progression in human gastric cancer. Oncology Reports. 2011;**25**:1271-1277. DOI: 10.3892/or.2011.1201

[112] Ljujic B, Radosavljevic G, Jovanovic I, Pavlovic S, Zdravkovic N, Milovanovic M, et al. Elevated serum level of IL-23 correlates with expression of VEGF in human colorectal carcinoma. Archives of Medical Research. 2010;**41**:182-189. DOI: 10.1016/j.arcmed.2010.02.009

[113] Radosavljevic G, Ljujic B, Jovanovic I, Srzentic Z, Pavlovic S, Zdravkovic N, et al. Interleukin-17 may be a valuable serum tumour marker in patients with colorectal carcinoma. Neoplasma. 2010;**57**:135-144. DOI: 10.4149/neo_2010_02_135

[114] Langowski JL, Zhang X, Wu L, Mattson JD, Chen T, Smith K, et al. IL-23 promotes tumour incidence and growth. Nature. 2006;**442**:46146-46145. DOI: 10.1038/nature04808

[115] Liang M, Liwen Z, Yun Z, Yanbo D, Jianping C. Serum levels of IL-33 and correlation with IL-4, IL-17A, and hypergammaglobulinemia in patients with autoimmune hepatitis. Mediators of Inflammation. 2018;**2018**:7964654. DOI: 10.1155/2018/7964654

[116] Pascual-Reguant A, Bayat Sarmadi J, Baumann C, Noster R, Cirera-Salinas D, Curato C, et al. TH17 cells express ST2 and are controlled by the alarmin IL-33 in the small intestine. Mucosal Immunology. 2017;**10**:1431-1442. DOI: 10.1038/mi.2017.5

[117] Cui G, Yuan A, Pang Z, Zheng W, Li Z, Goll R. Contribution of IL-33 to the pathogenesis of colorectal Cancer. Frontiers in Oncology. 2018;**8**:561. DOI: 10.3389/fonc.2018.00561

[118] Theoharides TC, Zhang B, Kempuraj D, Tagen M, Vasiadi M,

Angelidou A, et al. IL-33 augments substance P-induced VEGF secretion from human mast cells and is increased in psoriatic skin. Proceedings of the National Academy of Sciences of the United States of America. 2010;**107**:4448-4453. DOI: 10.1073/pnas.1000803107

[119] Choi YS, Choi HJ, Min JK, Pyun BJ, Maeng YS, Park H, et al. Interleukin-33 induces angiogenesis and vascular permeability through ST2/TRAF6-mediated endothelial nitric oxide production. Blood. 2009;**114**:3117-3126. DOI: 10.1182/blood-2009-02-203372

[120] Milosavljevic MZ, Jovanovic IP, Pejnovic NN, Mitrovic SL, Arsenijevic NN, Simovic Markovic BJ, et al. Deletion of IL-33R attenuates VEGF expression and enhances necrosis in mammary carcinoma. Oncotarget. 2016;**7**:18106-18115. DOI: 10.18632/oncotarget.7635

[121] Zhang Y, Davis C, Shah S, Hughes D, Ryan JC, Altomare D, et al. IL-33 promotes growth and liver metastasis of colorectal cancer in mice by remodeling the tumor microenvironment and inducing angiogenesis. Molecular Carcinogenesis. 2017;**56**:272-287. DOI: 10.1002/mc.22491

[122] Zhu WH, MacIntyre A, Nicosia RF. Regulation of angiogenesis by vascular endothelial growth factor and angiopoietin-1 in the rat aorta model: Distinct temporal patterns of intracellular signaling correlate with induction of angiogenic sprouting. The American Journal of Pathology. 2002;**161**:823-830. DOI: 10.1016/S0002-9440(10)64242-3

[123] Chung AS, Wu X, Zhuang G, Ngu H, Kasman I, Zhang J, et al. An interleukin-17-mediated paracrine network promotes tumor resistance to anti-angiogenic therapy. Nature Medicine. 2013;**19**:1114-1123. DOI: 10.1038/nm.3291

[124] Maniati E, Hagemann T. IL-17 mediates resistance to anti-VEGF therapy. Nature Medicine. 2013;**19**:1092-1094. DOI: 10.1038/nm.3333

[125] Rivera LB, Bergers G. Intertwined regulation of angiogenesis and immunity by myeloid cells. Trends in Immunology. 2015;**36**:240-249. DOI: 10.1016/j.it.2015.02.005

[126] Lu KV, Bergers G. Mechanisms of evasive resistance to anti-VEGF therapy in glioblastoma. CNS Oncology. 2013;**2**:49-65. DOI: 10.2217/cns.12.36

[127] de Oliveira JT, Ribeiro C, Barros R, Gomes C, de Matos AJ, Reis CA, et al. Hypoxia up-regulates Galectin-3 in mammary tumor progression and metastasis. PLoS One. 2015;**10**:e0134458. DOI: 10.1371/journal.pone.0134458

Chapter 6

Vascular Endothelial Growth Factor (VEGF) in Liver Disease

Darmadi Darmadi, Riska Habriel Ruslie and Cennikon Pakpahan

Abstract

Vascular endothelial growth factor (VEGF) is the most potent stimulating factor for angiogenesis. Its expression is related to inflammation and hypoxia. In normal conditions, VEGF is important in the wound healing process. The binding of VEGF with its receptors triggers angiogenesis and lymphangiogenesis and increases vascular permeability. Liver diseases comprise acute and chronic ones. Liver diseases cause inflammation and hypoxia, which increase VEGF level. If they occur chronically, persistent high VEGF levels will promote the risk of chronic liver diseases, including hepatic viral infections, alcoholic and nonalcoholic fatty liver diseases, liver cirrhosis, and finally hepatocellular carcinoma (HCC). High VEGF level is also associated with progressive disease course and poorer outcomes. Tissue remodeling by replacement of normal liver tissue with fibrous tissue occurs. Due to the importance of VEGF in angiogenesis and liver diseases, therapeutic agents targeting VEGF have been developed. Drugs that neutralize VEGF and modulate VEGF receptors have been approved for treating various disorders, including liver disease. Additionally, VEGF is a promising modality for diagnosing liver cirrhosis and HCC. VEGF may also be utilized to predict the outcome of the liver and to monitor the therapeutic response of patients.

Keywords: angiogenesis, carcinoma, cirrhosis, hepatocellular, liver, management, VEGF

1. Introduction

A hypothesis regarding blood vessel growth stimulating factors had been proposed nearly 70 years ago. This was based on the development of organs and diseases. The substance induces vessel growth in positive manner, such as normal retinal vasculature and negative ones, such as tumor cells [1]. In 1989, vascular endothelial growth factor (VEGF) was finally identified, isolated, and cloned [1, 2]. Gene coding human VEGF is located in chromosome 6p21.3. Its consists of 8 exons and is separated by seven introns [3, 4]. This structure makes a high genetic variation to become possible. Approximately 140 variations have been identified and affect the substance itself [4]. There are several subtypes of VEGF, including VEGF-A, VRGF-B, VEGF-C, VEGF-D, and placental growth factor (PlGF), with VEGF-A being the most frequently studied one. VEGF-A has isoforms, with the most common ones being VEGF-A_{121}, VEGF-A_{165},

VEGF-A_{189}, and VEGF-A_{165}. Each isoform has different heparin-binding ability. When VEGF binds its receptor, angiogenesis activity and vascular permeability are increased [1, 5–8]. VEFG also acts as an anti-apoptotic factor for endothelial cells, thus enhances angiogenesis [5, 7–9].

Liver cirrhosis represents the fate of almost all liver diseases. The prevalence of liver cirrhosis is estimated at 0.15% of the total population in USA. However, the exact prevalence is difficult to predict since many cases are asymptomatic. Liver cirrhosis is considered as a precursor for hepatic cellular carcinoma (HCC). HCC is one of the most common solid organ tumors globally [10] and the most common primary malignancy of the liver. It comprises approximately 80% of liver malignant lesions. Over 500,000 new cases are diagnosed annually worldwide. The incidence rate is increasing from time to time. In USA, the incidence had doubled from 1.4 per 100,000 in 1975–1977 to 4.8 per 100.000 in 2005–2007 [11]. Approximately 2 million deaths are recorded annually due to liver diseases. Half of them are caused by complications of liver cirrhosis and the rest is due to viral hepatitis and HCC. Liver cirrhosis and HCC account for 3.5% of global deaths. In developed countries, liver cirrhosis is most commonly caused by alcohol and non-alcoholic fatty liver (NAFLD) while hepatitis B is the most common etiology of liver cirrhosis in China, other Asian, and African countries [10–12]. Liver cirrhosis and HCC are the third most common cause of death in European countries. The overall 5-year survival is less than 12%. Both conditions also increase the rate of liver transplantation [5, 10, 11]. In USA, chronic liver disease-related hospitalization is constantly increased from 3056 in 2012 to 3757 in 2016 per 100,000 cases with total inpatient hospitalization costs increased from $14.9 billion to $18.8 billion. Among all chronic liver diseases, alcoholic and non-alcoholic fatty liver diseases are dominant with an increasing trend. The presence of liver cirrhosis and HCC further worsens the socioeconomic burden of chronic liver diseases [13].

Liver cirrhosis and HCC progression are associated with angiogenesis. Angiogenesis increases hepatic resistance and the risk of liver failure, leading to manifestations such as gastroesophageal varices, upper gastrointestinal bleeding, ascites, spontaneous bacterial peritonitis, and hepatic encephalopathy. Angiogenesis also plays a critical role in HCC growth and metastases. VEGF is the main pro-angiogenic factor in the liver. Its expression is increased in pathological conditions of the liver. The underlying triggers such as hypoxia, inflammation, and mechanical stress have been proven to increase VEGF levels in liver diseases [2]. In this article, we will discuss VEGF mechanism of action, its role in liver diseases, and its importance in the management of liver diseases.

2. Mechanism of action of VEGF

Hypoxia and inflammation are the most frequent triggers for VEGF production. Inflammation exerts tissue damage and activates endothelial cells. Both conditions triggers VEGF production in concordance with the tissue repair mechanism. Hypoxia itself may trigger VEGF production by the role of hypoxia-inducible factors (HIF). Hypoxia also triggers further inflammation and creates a viscous cycle between inflammation and angiogenesis [14, 15]. VEGF binds to its receptor with the aid of neuropilins as co-receptor and activates tyrosine kinase. There are three subtypes of VEGF receptor and binding of VEGF-A elicits the most potent signaling for angiogenesis (**Figure 1**). The receptors are found in a wide variety of cell types

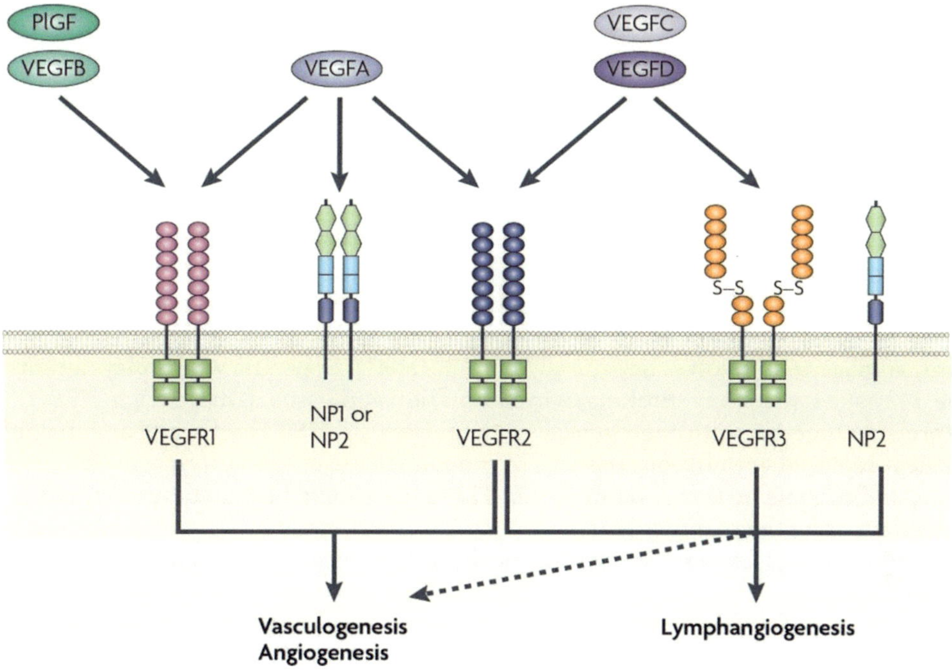

Figure 1.
Binding of VEGF subtypes with VEGF receptor subtypes elicits various processes including angiogenesis. PlGF: Placental growth factor, VEGF: Vascular endothelial growth factor, NP: Neuropilin [6].

including endothelial cell, hematopoietic stem cell, monocyte, macrophage, and lymphatic endothelial cell. Tyrosine kinase then activates the signaling pathway through mediators such as phosphatidylinositol kinase, mitogen-activated kinase, and protein kinase C. These mediators promote angiogenesis, lymphangiogenesis, and vascular permeability, accordingly [2, 6, 8, 15, 16]. Nitric oxide is the first substance produced after binding between VEGF and its receptor. The later process increases intracellular calcium, activates calmodulin, and increases NO synthesis. Elevated NO is in line with increased vascular permeability and endothelial cell survival [2, 14]. The extravasation of vascular content including extracellular matrix components marks the initial angiogenesis process. Endothelial cell proliferation, tube formation, and branching of new vessels will occur. When the repair mechanism is completed, angiogenesis will be stopped by the action of inhibitors such as plasminogen activator inhibitors [14]. Overall, angiogenesis is regulated by a balance between stimulating and inhibiting factors [8].

3. VEGF and liver disease

Angiogenesis is a process of new blood vessel formation. As blood vessels carry important nutrients to organs and dispose of unnecessary metabolites, angiogenesis plays important homeostatic role [1, 14]. In normal conditions, angiogenesis is important in liver regeneration from several conditions including partial hepatectomy and liver transplantation [5, 17]. This is called physiological angiogenesis and involves liver sinusoidal endothelial cells. The process starts at 48–72 hours after the damage and peaking at 4–5 days. Angiogenesis may occur from pre-existing blood vessels or directly from endothelial cell proliferation [5, 9].

Unregulated angiogenesis causes a negative impact and results in diseases including tumors. Unregulated angiogenesis may result from an imbalance between pro- and anti-angiogenesis. In this situation, VEGF is the culprit. Several abnormalities regarding VEGF coding genes are one of the underlying pathogenesis of the diseases [1, 5, 17]. Baitello et al. conducted a study to determine the role of genetic variations in liver disease, particularly HCC. They observed that VEGF polymorphism C936T and A1154G are associated with elevated VEGF level and incidence of HCC [18]. VEGF promotes angiogenesis and increases vascular permeability. Tissue hypoxia is the major signaling for VEGF expression [1, 5, 17]. In liver, angiogenesis involves hepatic stellate cell (HSC), a specific which plays a central role in tissue remodeling. Prolonged inflammation and tissue damage trigger VEGF expression together with angiogenesis. In angiogenesis, HSC is activated and normal tissue is replaced with fibrous tissue. This impairs tissue oxygenation, cerates hypoxia state, and triggers further inflammation. This cycle should be halted by eliminating any points from the pathway [14].

Elevated VEGF level is proposed in alcoholic liver disease. Luo et al. investigated liver tissue of rats with alcoholic liver disease. They found that mRNA level of VEGF is elevated significantly in liver tissue of rats with the alcoholic liver disease compared to liver tissue of normal rats. A similar finding was reported for mRNA level of HIF. The degree of disease was positively correlated with VEGF and HIF mRNA levels. The trigger of VEGF overexpression, in this case, is different from other liver diseases. In alcoholic liver disease, VEGF overexpression is triggered by leptin that is released from adipocytes [14, 19]. Kasztelan-Szczerbinska et al. confirmed the previous study. The level of plasma VEGF in patients with alcoholic liver disease in their study is significantly higher compared to healthy control [15]. Serum VEGF level may also distinguish between alcoholic liver disease and chronic hepatic viral infections. A higher level was observed in alcoholic liver disease. However, further studies are mandatory before extrapolating this result in general population [20]. Similar to nonalcoholic fatty liver disease (NAFLD), the expression of VEGF is up-regulated by a different pathway. Leptin as an adipocytokine plays a central role in promoting VEGF and other pro-inflammatory cytokines expression. VEGF expression is elevated through the recruitment and stabilization of HIF by leptin. This leads to angiogenesis and fibrogenesis, and progression from NAFLD to non-alcoholic steatohepatitis (NASH) [14, 17]. The severity of steatosis in NASH is associated positively with VEGF level [17].

Pathological angiogenesis has been observed in chronic liver diseases for a long period of time. This phenomenon is observed in chronic hepatitis B and C, autoimmune hepatitis, and primary biliary cirrhosis. The damage suffered by the liver triggers inflammation and initiates the wound healing process with increased expression of several growth factors including VEGF. Elevated VEGF level promotes angiogenesis then angiogenesis leads to fibrosis and liver tissue remodeling distinctive of liver cirrhosis. The latter process involves hepatic stellate cells which produce an extracellular matrix. If the damage occurs chronically, high VEGF expression also becomes chronic, followed by chronic angiogenesis and fibrogenesis. Hypoxia resulted from extensive fibrogenesis further increases VEGF expression as stated above, which is mediated by HIF. Lately, it is found that not only VEGF level is increased but also VEGF receptor [5, 14, 17]. Hepatitis B virus itself surprisingly can induce VEGF release without the presence of inflammation and hypoxia state. The positive correlation is reported between serum VEGF level and severity of chronic liver diseases [14].

A study by Franchitto et al. supports the previous facts. Patients with chronic viral hepatitis and primary biliary cirrhosis have abundant hepatic progenitor cells in their liver. Furthermore, VEGF and its receptor's expression is increased in those progenitor cells. The number of progenitor cells expressing VEGF is correlated with angiogenesis, fibrogenesis, and carcinogenesis in subjects in their study [21]. VEGF is level not only elevated in primary liver disease but also in diseases with liver complications. Nihei, et al. conducted a study in children with Kawasaki disease. They found that inflammatory growth factors are elevated in all patients. More than half of the patients in their study had liver dysfunction as a complication from Kawasaki disease and VEGF was significantly elevated in patients with liver dysfunction compared to those without liver dysfunction [22].

Massive formation of portosystemic collateral vessels particularly in the esophagus and gut is the underlying pathogenesis of variceal bleeding. Collateral vessels shunt blood from portal to systemic circulation and cause substances that are normally detoxified by the liver to enter the systemic circulation. This leads to encephalopathy and sepsis in patients with liver disease. VEGF also contributes to portal hypertension. Angiogenesis increases blood flow in splanchnic organs draining into the portal vein and further increases portal venous flow. Nitic oxide furtherly enhances vasodilatation and blood flow. VEGF is known to promote nitric oxide level [5, 14, 17, 23]. Tissue remodeling also increases liver tissue resistance and ends with portal hypertension [14]. An animal study conducted by Huang et al. shows that rats with portal hypertension have increased VEGF expression as high as 40% compared to healthy rats as control. Portal pressure was also positively correlated with VEGF level [23]. Spider angiomas also result from elevated VEGF level. A study proved that subjects with liver cirrhosis and spider angiomas have higher plasma VEGF level compared to liver cirrhotic patients without spider angiomas [24].

Liver cirrhosis is the end-point of chronic liver disease and predisposing lesion to HCC. Chronic damage to liver maintains a high VEGF level over time and is associated with continuous angiogenesis and fibrogenesis. In the end, liver tissue is replaced by abnormal fibrous tissue [12]. Li et al. reported that plasma VEGF level is elevated significantly in liver cirrhotic patients compared to control group [24]. Abdelmoaty et al. also conducted a study regarding serum VEGF level in patients with liver cirrhosis. Serum VEGF level was significantly increased in patients with liver cirrhosis compared to healthy individuals. This result is in line with the result from previous study. Serum VEGF level was also positively related to degree of liver dysfunction based on Child-pugh score [25].

In cancers, increased expression of VEGF is positively associated with its growth and risk of metastases but negatively associated with the outcome of disease. VEGF triggers angiogenesis and angiogenesis itself nurtures the cancer cells [1, 6–8]. HCC is a highly vascularized cancer thus its progression and outcome are closely related to angiogenesis [5, 21, 26, 27]. Additionally, VEGF acts in an autocrine fashion in HCC. A study by Sharma et al. showed that both VEGF and its receptor expressions are elevated in HCC cell lines. This marks the ability of cancer tissue to grow independently from normal angiogenesis pathway [28]. The high angiogenesis activity in HCC is suspected due to increased oxygen demand by cancer cells during their growth trigger hypoxia state. Hypoxia further increases pro-angiogenesis factors including VEGF. VEGF has a good discrimination ability between HCC and chronic liver diseases. Therefore, it can be utilized as one of the diagnostic modality to detect HCC at its early stage [8]. Li et al. conducted a study in patients with HCC, benign liver lesions, and normal controls. The result showed that plasma VEGF level in HCC patients is significantly elevated compared to patients with benign liver lesions and normal subjects. In HCC group itself, subjects with large tumor size, distant metastasis, portal vein thrombosis, and arterial-portal vein shunting had higher plasma VEGF level compared to their counterparts [29]. The above result is confirmed by Zhang et al. In their study, plasma VEGF level was higher in HCC patients with multiple lesions, lesion larger than 5 cm, bilobar tumor distribution, and metastasized cancer [30]. In contrast, Uematsu et al. found different results in their study. Serum VEGF level was increased in patients with HCC and significantly higher compared to healthy volunteers but the difference was not significant if being compared with liver cirrhosis [27].

4. VEGF and management of liver disease

As HCC possesses high morbidity and mortality rates, diagnosis at its early stage is important to improve the patient's outcome. Hamdy et al. reported that VEGF is a promising diagnostic modality for HCC from their study. A VEGF cut off point of ≥280 pg./mL has sensitivity of 60.27% and specificity of 100% in discriminating HCC and chronic liver diseases from healthy subjects while a cutoff point of ≥482 pg./mL has sensitivity of 52.59% and specificity of 100% in discriminating HCC from chronic liver diseases [26]. Mukozu et al. in their study also proposed VEGF as novel marker for HCC diagnosis in patients with chronic hepatitis C virus infection. They reported that serum VEGF is better compared to alpha-fetoprotein in discriminating between HCC and liver cirrhosis. The sensitivity and specificity of VEGF were reported to be 98% and 46%, respectively. The values were obtained with a VEGF cutoff of 108 pg./mL [31]. Jinno et al. supported the previous findings. They proved that plasma VEGF level in subjects with HCC is significantly higher compared to healthy control, subjects with chronic hepatitis, and subjects with liver cirrhosis. Furthermore, plasma VEGF level in stage IV-B HCC patients was significantly higher among all stage groups. This implies that besides diagnosing HCC, VEGF is also useful in diagnosing metastasized HCC [32]. Another study from Japan reported concordance results. Serum VEGF level is higher in advanced HCC such as stage IV-B disease, giant and multinodular lesion, and distant metastasized disease [20].

Considering the role of VEGF in liver diseases, management focusing on VEGF manipulation has become popular [1, 5, 33]. Judah Folkman had hypothesized a strategy for managing cancers and other diseases with anti-angiogenesis [1]. The strategy comprises VEGF, its receptors, and it signaling pathways interventions. Nowadays, there are drugs targeting VEGF such as bevacizumab, ziv-aflibercept, rapamycin, and ramucirumab [1, 2, 5–7]. Bevacizumab and ramucirumab are neutralizing antibodies to VEGF. Approved in 2004, bevacizumab has become the most widely used anti-VEGF in the field of oncology. Ziv-aflibercept is soluble VEGF receptor that prevents the binding of VEGF with its natural receptor [1, 2, 6, 7].

Other agents such as tyrosine kinase receptor inhibitors (sunitinib, sorafenib, and imatinib) have been approved as therapeutic agents [5, 7, 33]. Among all, sorafenib which was developed in 1990 has become the most commonly used agent for HCC treatment [33]. The list of anti-angiogenic agents may be observed in **Table 1** [2]. In

Agents	Mechanism of action	Approved by FDA
Bevacizumab, ramucirumab	Monoclonal antibody against VEGF	Yes
Ziv-aflibercept	Decoy VEGF receptor	Yes
Sorafenib, sunitinib, apatinib, axitinib, cabozantinib, lenvatinib, nintedanib, pazopanib, regorafinib, imantinib	Tyrosine kinase inhibitor	Yes
Cediranib, lucitanib, semaxanib, tivozanib	Tyrosine kinase inhibitor	No

FDA: Food and Drug Administration, VEGF: vascular endothelial growth factor.

Table 1.
List of anti-angiogenesis agents and their mechanism of action [2, 6].

vivo studies proved that the agent may decrease pathologic angiogenesis as high as 52% in patients with liver diseases. Combination with other anti-angiogenesis agent is also urged and shows better outcome in patients. Platelet-derived growth factor (PDGF) signaling inhibitor is one of the treatment modality in the combination regime [5].

Single anti-angiogenesis therapy is effective in several cancers including HCC in the advanced stage [7]. Some side effects should be put in consideration when administering anti-angiogenesis therapy. Hypertension, renal dysfunction, proteinuria, thrombosis, bleeding, and arrhythmia are the most common side effects reported. Hypertension is the most common side effect, occurring in 25% of patients treated with anti-angiogenesis. This is strongly related with decreased NO level due to anti-angiogenesis agents. Similar mechanisms underlie further side effects [2, 6]. Resistance against anti-angiogenesis therapy is another threatening problem even though this phenomenon has not been proven consistently. However, long-term follow-up showed the tendency of growing resistance to this treatment [6].

Serum VEGF level is also useful in monitoring a patient's response toward therapies. Matsui et al. measured serum VEGF level in patients with HCC receiving chemotherapy. The chemotherapeutic agents used were leucovorin, cisplatin, and 5-fluorouracil. The results showed that serum VEGF level is higher in patients with partial response or stable disease compared to progressive disease [20]. A similar result is reported by Li et al. Even though the treatment modality in their study was different (transcatheter arterial chemoembolization/TACE), the result showed that patients with high pre-therapeutic plasma VEGF level are associated with poor response to treatment [29]. Plasma VEGF level is suggested to be a modality for monitoring prognosis after liver transplantation in HCC cases. A plasma VEGF level of >44 pg/mL is associated with worse overall and disease-free survival. Additionally, it is also associated with higher disease recurrence and poorer disease outcomes [30]. However, an anomaly was submitted by Shigesawa et al. They observed HCC patients receiving anti-angiogenesis agent for 8 weeks and found that serum VEGF level is significantly lower in patients who experienced deterioration compared to those without deterioration [34]. Ramadan et al. found similar result with Shigesawa et al. Patients with hepatitis C virus-associated HCC had higher VEGF level after receiving treatments compared to those untreated ones. The recurrence rate became higher in line with elevated VEGF level [16]. These findings raise suspicion regarding the possibility of treatment resistance.

5. Conclusions

Liver diseases are conditions that may occur both acutely or chronically. Liver cirrhosis and HCC are the end-points of chronic liver diseases which carry heavy socioeconomic burden. Angiogenesis plays a significant role in liver diseases, including alcoholic fatty liver disease, NAFLD, chronic hepatic viral infections, and their progressions. The most potent mediator for angiogenesis is VEGF. A high level of VEGF is associated with an increased incidence of liver disease and a worse clinical course. Inflammation and hypoxia from chronic liver diseases are the triggering factors for VEGF release. The binding of VEGF with its receptors triggers angiogenesis, lymphangiogenesis, and vascular permeability increment. If occur for a long period, liver tissue remodeling is observed as a precursor lesion of HCC. Due to the importance of angiogenesis, anti-angiogenesis therapy targeting VEGF is becoming popular. Several agents that neutralize VEGF and modulate its receptors have been approved to treat various diseases. Besides, VEGF is also a promising modality for the diagnosis of liver diseases and for predicting disease outcomes. The therapeutic response of patients may also be monitored using VEGF level.

Conflict of interest

The authors declare no conflict of interest.

Author details

Darmadi Darmadi[1*], Riska Habriel Ruslie[2] and Cennikon Pakpahan[3]

1 Faculty of Medicine, Department of Internal Medicine, Universitas Sumatera Utara, Medan, Indonesia

2 Faculty of Medicine, Department of Child Health, Universitas Prima Indonesia, Medan, Indonesia

3 Faculty of Medicine, Department of Biomedical Sciences, Universitas Airlangga, Surabaya, Indonesia

*Address all correspondence to: darmadi@usu.ac.id

References

[1] Apte RS, Chen DS, Ferrara N. VEGF in signaling and disease: Beyond discovery and development. Cell. 2019;**176**:1248-1264. DOI: 10.1016/j.cell.2019.01.021

[2] Pandey AK, Singhi EK, Arroyo JP, Ikizler TA, Gould ER, Brown J, et al. Mechanisms of VEGF (vascular endothelial growth factor) inhibitor-associated hypertension and vascular disease. Hypertension. 2018;**71**:e1-e8. DOI: 10.1161/HYPERTENSIONAHA.117.10271

[3] Sa-Nguanraksa D, O-Charoenrat P. The role of vascular endothelial growth factor a polymorphisms in breast cancer. International Journal of Molecular Sciences. 2012;**13**:14845-14864. DOI: 10.3390/ijms131114845

[4] Jain L, Vargo CA, Danesi R, Sissung TM, Price DK, Venzon D, et al. The role of vascular endothelial growth factor SNPs as predictive and prognostic markers for major solid tumors. Molecular Cancer Therapeutics. 2009;**8**:2496-2508. DOI: 10.1158/1535-7163.mct-09-0302

[5] Fernandez M, Semela D, Bruix J, Colle I, Pinzani M, Bosch J. Angiogeneis in liver disease. Journal of Hepatology. 2009;**50**:604-620. DOI: 10.1016/j.jhep.2008.12.011

[6] Shibuya M. Vascular endothelial growth factor (VEGF) and its receptor (VEGFR) signaling in angiogenesis. Genes & Cancer. 2011;**2**:1097-1105. DOI: 10.1177/1947601911423031

[7] Ellis L, Hicklin D. VRGF-targeted therapy: Mechanism of anti-tumour activity. Nature Reviews. Cancer. 2008;**8**:579-591. DOI: 10.1038/ncr2403

[8] Karamysheva AF. Mechanism of angiogenesis. Biochemistry (Mosc). 2008;**73**:751-762. DOI: 10.1134/s0006297908070031

[9] Lu J, Zhao Y, Zhang X, Li L. The vascular endothelial growth factor signaling pathway regulates liver sinusoidal epithelial cells during liver regeneration after partial hepatectomy. Expert Review of Gastroenterology & Hepatology. 2021;**15**:139-147. DOI: 10.1080/17474124.2020.1815532

[10] Asrani SK, Devarbhavi H, Eaton J, Kamath PS. Burden of liver diseases in the world. Journal of Hepatology. 2019;**70**:151-171. DOI: 10.1016/j.jhep.2018.09.014

[11] Mittal S, El-Serag HB. Epidemiology of HCC: Consider the population. Journal of Clinical Gastroenterology. 2013;**47**:S2-S6. DOI: 10.1097/MCG.0b013e3182872f29

[12] Schuppan D, Afdhal NH. Liver cirrhosis. Lancet. 2008;**371**:838-851. DOI: 10.1016/S0140-6736(08)60383-9

[13] Hirode G, SAAb S, Wong RJ. Trends in the burden of chronic liver disease among hospitalized US adults. JAMA Network Open. 2020;**3**:e201997. DOI: 10.1001/jamanetworkopen.2020.1997

[14] Elpek GO. Angiogenesis and liver fibrosis. World Journal of Hepatology. 2015;7:377-391. DOI: 10.4254/wjh.v7.i3.377

[15] Kasztelan-Szczerbinska B, Surdacka A, Slomka M, Rolinski J, Celinski K, Cichoz-Lach H, et al. Angiogenesis-related biomarkers in patients with alcoholic liver disease: Their association with liver disease

complications and outcome. Mediators of Inflammation. 2014;**2014**:673032. DOI: 10.1155/2014/673032

[16] Ramadan HK, Meghezel EM, Abdel-Malek MO, Askar AA, Hetta HF, Mahmoud AA, et al. Correlation between vascular endothelial growth factor and long-term occurrence of HCV-related hepatocellular carcinoma after treatment with direct-acting antivirals. Cancer Investigation. 2021;**39**:653-660. DOI: 10.1080/07357907.2021.1951751

[17] Bocca C, Novo E, Miglietta A, Parola M. Angiogenesis and fibrosis in chronic liver diseases. Cellular and Molecular Gastroenterology and Hepatology. 2015;**1**:477-488. DOI: 10.1016/j.jcmgh.2015.06.011

[18] Baitello MEL, Tenani GD, Ferreira RF, Nogueira V, Pinhel MAS, da Silva RCMA, et al. VEGF polymorphisms related to higher serum levels of protein identify patients with hepatocellular carcinoma. Canadian Journal of Gastroenterology & Hepatology. 2016;**2016**:9607054. DOI: 10.1155/2016/9607054

[19] Luo R, Yi Z, Wu W, Meng W. The mRNA levels of PPARα, HIF-1α, and VEGF in liver tissues of rats with alcoholic liver disease. American Journal of Translational Research. 2021;**13**:11932-11937

[20] Matsui D, Nagai H, Mukozo T, Ogino YU, Sumino Y. VEGF in patients with advanced hepatocellular carcinoma receiving intra-arterial chemotherapy. Anticancer Research. 2015;**35**:2205-2210

[21] Franchitto A, Onori P, Renzi A, Carpino G, Mancinelli R, Alvaro D, et al. Expression of vascular endothelial growth factors and their receptors by hepatic progenitor cells in human liver diseases. Hepatobiliary Surgery and Nutrition. 2013;**2**:68-77. DOI: 10.3978/j.issn.2304-3881.2012.10.11

[22] Nihei K, Ikeda C, Hosono T, Aoki T, Shinomiya N. Effect of the vascular endothelial growth factor (VEGF) on liver dysfunction in the acute phase of Kawasaki disease. Pediatric Research. 2003;**53**:171. DOI: 10.1203/00006450-200301000-00108

[23] Huang H, Haq O, Utsumi T, Sethasine S, Abraldes JG, Groszmann RJ, et al. Intestinal and plasma VEGF levels in cirrhosis: The role of portal pressure. Journal of Cellular and Molecular Medicine. 2012;**16**:1125-1133. DOI: 10.1111/j.1582-4934.2011.01399.x

[24] Li C, Lee F, Hwang S, Lu R, Lee W, Chao Y, et al. Spider angiomas in patients with liver cirrhosis: Role of vascular endothelial growth factor and basic fibroblast growth factor. World Journal of Gastroenterology. 2003;**9**:2832-2835. DOI: 10.3748/wjg.v9.i12.2832

[25] Abdelmoaty MA, Bogdady AM, Attia MM, Zaky NA. Circulating vascular endothelial growth factor and nitric oxide in patients with liver cirrhosis: A possible association with liver function impairment. Indian Journal of Clinical Biochemistry. 2009;**24**:398-403. DOI: 10.1007/s12291-009-0071-5

[26] Hamdy MN, Shaheen KY, Awad MAM, Barakat EMF, Shalaby SI, Gupta N, et al. Vascular endothelial growth factor (VEGF) as a biochemical marker for the diagnosis of hepatocellular carcinoma (HCC). Clinics and Practice. 2020;**17**:1441-1453

[27] Uematsu S, Higashi T, Nouso K, Kariyama K, Nakamura S, Suzuki M, et al. Altered expression of vascular endothelial growth factor, fibroblast growth factor-2 and endostatin in patients with hepatocellular carcinoma.

Journal of Gastroenterology and Hepatology. 2005;**20**:583-588. DOI: 10.1111/j.1440-1746.2005.03726.x

[28] Sharma BK, Srinivasan R, Chawla YK, Chakraborti A. Vascular endothelial growth factor: Evidence for autocrine signaling in hepatocellular carcinoma cell lines affecting invasion. Indian Journal of Cancer. 2016;**53**:542-547. DOI: 10.4103/0019-509X.204765

[29] Li X, Feng G, Zheng C, Zhuo C, Liu X. Expression of plasma vascular endothelial growth factor in patients with hepatocellular carcinoma and effect of transcatheter arterial chemoembolization therapy on plasma vascular endothelial growth factor level. World Journal of Gastroenterology. 2004;**10**:2878-2882. DOI: 10.3748/wjg/v10.i19.2878

[30] Zhang W, Kim R, Quintini C, Hashimoto K, Fujiki M, Diago T, et al. Prognostic role of plasma vascular endothelial growth factor in patients with hepatocellular carcinoma undergoing liver transplantation. Liver Transplantation. 2015;**21**:101-111. DOI: 10.1002/lt.24013

[31] Mukozu T, Nagai H, Matsui, Kanekawa T, Sumino Y. Serum VEGF as a tumor marker in patients with HCV-related liver cirhhosis and hepatocellular carcinoma. Anticancer Research. 2013;**33**:1031-1021

[32] Jinno K, Tanimizu M, Hyodo I, Nishikawa Y, Hosokawa Y, Doi T, et al. Circulating vascular endothelial growth factor (VEGF) is a possible tumor marker for metastasis in human hepatocellular carcinoma. Journal of Gastroenterology. 1988;**33**:376-382. DOI: 10.1007/s005350050099

[33] Daher S, Massarwa M, Benson AA, Khoury T. Current and future treatment of hepatocellular carcinoma: An updated comprehensive review. Journal of Clinical and Translational Hepatology. 2017;**6**:69-78. DOI: 10.14218/JCTH.2017.00031

[34] Shigesawa T, Suda G, Kimura M, Maehara O, Tokuchi Y, Kubo A, et al. Baseline serum angiopoietin-2 and VEGF levels predict the deterioration of the liver functional reserve during levantinib treatment for hepatocellular carcinoma. PLoS One. 2021;**16**:e0247728. DOI: 10.1371/journal.pone.0247728

Chapter 7

Adipocytokines: Are They the Theory of Cancer Progression?

Rowyda Nawwaf Al-Harithy

Abstract

Adipocytokines have gained significant attention in the scientific community over the past few decades. They are a family of enzymes, hormones, growth factors, proteins, and other bioactive molecules that are important regulators of many processes. Adipocytokines are predominantly produced by preadipocytes and mature adipocytes to act through a network of autocrine, paracrine, and endocrine pathways. Leptin (LEP) is the first adipocytokine discovered that has a role in modulating adiposity and has been shown to exert pleiotropic effects on many metabolic pathways through the leptin receptors (LEPRs). LEP has pro-tumoral roles; it promotes angiogenesis, proliferation, survival of tumor cells, and inhibits apoptosis. To exercise its role in tumorigenesis, LEP-LEPR signaling and epithelial-mesenchymal transitions (EMTs) play a significant role. LEP is an oncogenic factor mainly due to its proinflammatory and proangiogenic effects. In angiogenesis, LEP acts directly as an endothelial growth factor or indirectly through cellular pathways, such as STAT3/ERK1/2, JAK2/STAT3, MAPK/ERK, PI3K/AKT, p38, p53, MAPK, and Wnt/β-catenin.

Keywords: adipocytokines, leptin, inflammation, angiogenesis, cancer

1. Introduction

Adipose tissue is a complex, dynamic, and heterogenic endocrine organ with diverse homeostatic processes [1]. During the past few decades, the structural and functional principles of adipose tissue have evolved considerably to get to today's concept [2]. In the human body, the adipose tissue is restricted in depot sites and varies in cellular composition and character. Adipose tissue can be classified by morphology into white, brown, beige, pink, and yellow [3]. Our understanding of their importance started with identifying a range of adipose tissue products and their functions. Since then, much has been learned about how adipose tissue communicates with other organs of the body. More recently, its functions have been reported to be highly influenced by bioactive molecules with widespread systemic effects contributing to numerous physiological and pathological processes [4]. The white adipose depots are considered a specialized organ representing the largest endocrine tissue in humans. It can be broadly classified by location into subcutaneous and visceral. In its different locations, it shows different metabolic profiles with different functions. In general, they are responsible for storing chemical energy formatted as triglycerides packed in unilocular lipid droplets. The white adipocytes, especially in the visceral area, secrete

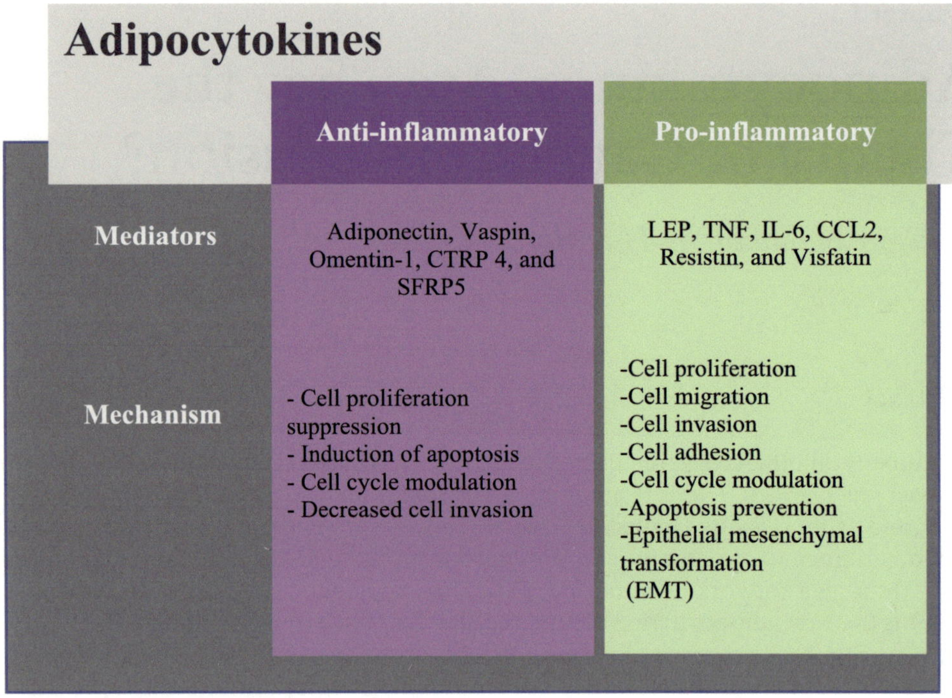

Figure 1.
Adipocytokines and their mechanisms as an anti-inflammatory and proinflammatory.

abundant mediators, including exosomes, miRNA, lipids, inflammatory cytokines, and peptide hormones that participate in the process of interorgan communication via paracrine and endocrine modes [5].

White adipose tissue comprises many different cell types; approximately 40–50% of the cells are adipocytes, with the rest represented by the stromal vascular fraction (SVF) of cells, including preadipocytes, fibroblasts cells, endothelial cells, vascular progenitor cells, mesenchymal stem cells, and a variety of immune cells (macrophages, natural killer cells, B-lymphocytes, and T-lymphocytes) [6]. Adipocytes, specific to white adipose tissue, are plastic and respond to changes in metabolism by altering their size, number, and their exerted functions [7, 8]. The white adipose tissue multifarious composition renders white adipose tissue an important mediator of metabolism and inflammation [9]. White adipose tissue influences metabolism through maintaining energy homeostasis, adipocyte differentiation, and insulin sensitivity. It also affects inflammation through its actions in the immune system as pro- and anti-inflammatory mediators (**Figure 1**). This function is controlled by numerous adipocytokines, other cytokines, chemokines, and growth factors [10]. While the term adipokine is commonly used to refer to adipose tissue-derived proteins, adipocytokines are mainly, but not solely, produced by adipocytes.

2. Adipocytokines

The word adipocytokine is derived from the Greek root meaning fat cell movement. Adipocytokines are produced exclusively or substantially by preadipocytes and mature adipocytes, hence their name. They are biologically active molecules that are important regulators for many physiological processes. Adipocytokines are heterogeneous in structure and function, which is mainly affected by the specific anatomical location of the producing adipocytes. Adipocytokines have the ability to act locally or distally as inflammatory, immune, or hormonal signalers. They can be categorized in terms of their function as metabolic factors, proinflammatory factors, proangiogenic factors, and extracellular matrix components. Adipocytokines are secreted in response to different triggers; their involvement has been noted in insulin action, endothelial cell function, blood pressure, appetite, hemostasis, reproduction, angiogenesis, and immunity [11].

The year 2022 marks the 35th anniversary of adipocytokines. The breakthrough discovery of the first adipocytokine, adipsin, followed by tumor necrosis factor (TNF), leptin (LEP), and adiponectin led to the widespread recognition of adipose tissue as an endocrine organ. Adipsin (also known as complement factor D) was identified as an adipokine in 1987 [12]. In 1993, TNF was identified as a proinflammatory adipocytokine in the models of diabetes and obesity, becoming pioneering evidence for a functional link between obesity and inflammation [13]. The identification and cloning of LEP in 1994 followed by that of adiponectin in 1995 were an inflection point into the endocrine era [14, 15]. LEP and adiponectin are the classic adipocytokines of visceral adipose tissue and clearly the two most widely studied adipocyte products. LEP is acknowledged as an adipose tissue-specific secreted protein that regulates food intake and energy. Adiponectin, also known as ACRP30, AdipoQ, and gelatin-binding protein-28, has anti-inflammatory actions on the liver, the heart, the kidneys, muscle cells, and pancreatic β cells, to name a few [16–18]. It plays roles that are most likely relevant to cognitive dysfunction, namely, synaptic regulation, insulin sensitivity, neuroinflammation, neuroprotection, and neurogenesis [19, 20].

Adiponectin and LEP's detailed mechanisms of action at the cellular level of their target organs and their mutual effects on each other remain ambiguous. Despite extensive research on the topic, much more regarding LEP and adiponectin, their relationship to each other and to the body remains to be discovered. However, it is important to note that the ratio of adiponectin to LEP has been proposed as a marker of adipose tissue dysfunction [21, 22]. On review of the literature, LEP is found to be the most studied in the context of cancer risk and progression (**Figure 1**).

3. Leptin

Friedman and his colleagues discovered LEP in 1994 and named it after the word "leptos," which means thin in Greek reference to its demonstrated effect on the body. In humans, LEP is encoded by the LEP gene that is located on chromosome 7 7q31.3 and consists of three exonic regions with two intronic regions. It is a nonglycosylated adipocytokine consisting of 146 amino acids. LEP is a multifunctional adipocytokine primarily secreted by the white adipocytes. LEP is also produced by other tissues, such as the stomach, placenta, and mammary glands [23–26]. The past 25 years of research on LEP have provided important insights into the intricate network that links nutrition, metabolism, reproduction, endocrine regulation, inflammation, and immune function [27–29]. LEP is a key regulator of the adipose organ, and its main task is to regulate energy balance, which is possible by lowering the appetite. The essential characteristics of LEP are listed in **Table 1**.

Adipocytokine	Characteristics
Leptin (LEP)	Signals through leptin receptor isoform b (LEPRb)
	Binds short and soluble leptin receptor isoforms (LEPRa, LEPRc)
	Regulates bone mass
	Regulates reproduction
	Regulates body weight gain
	Regulates immune cell functions
	Regulates food intake and energy expenditure
	Regulates glucose tolerance and insulin sensitivity
	Regulates brain sympathetic output to different tissues
	May regulate body temperature
	May regulate hematopoiesis
	Induce epithelial-mesenchymal transition
	Promote adipogenesis
	Increases adipocyte lipolysis
	Increases angiogenesis
	Increases brown adipose tissue activity
	Increases skeletal muscle cell glucose uptake
	Increases adipocyte, hepatocyte, and skeletal muscle cell fatty acid oxidation
	May increase adipose tissue stromal cell proliferation
	May increase white adipose tissue browning
	Decreases adipocyte glucose uptake
	Decreases adipocyte, hepatocyte, and skeletal muscle cell lipogenesis

Table 1.
The functions of leptin.

LEP expression in the adipose tissue is influenced by a variety of hormones, including insulin, glucocorticoids, catecholamines, and cortisol, and several other metabolic factors, including TNF-α, fatty acids, and glucose [30–33]. Recently, a fat-specific long noncoding RNA (lncRNA) has been identified to interact with redundant enhancers and regulate LEP expression [34]. LEP deficiency or resistance is associated with the dysregulation of cytokine production, increased susceptibility to infections, autoimmune disorders, malnutrition, and inflammatory responses. The elevated levels of serum LEP have been unequivocally correlated with an increased risk of developing various tumor forms, including testicular, breast, prostate, colon, and pancreatic cancers [35–40]. The short-, medium-, and long-term regulatory actions of LEP are supported by its specific LEP receptor (LEPR). The LEPR is a class I cytokine receptor and structurally a transmembrane receptor encoded by the *LEPR* (*OBR*) gene on chromosome 1p31.3 [41–43]. In humans, there are at least four splice variants of the LEPR gene that have been identified and categorized as long (LEPRb), short (LEPRa, and LEPRc), and secretive (LEPRe) isoforms. The isoforms have different lengths of intracellular C-terminal domains. The LEPRb contains the full intracellular domain 303 amino acids, and the short isoforms contain 32–40 amino acids. Although long and short isoforms share a sequence of 29 amino acids proximal to the transmembrane region, the LEPRe isoform lacks both transmembrane and cytoplasmic domains [44, 45]. The long LEPR contains the full intracellular domain to fully induce intracellular signaling necessary for the activation of critical second messenger pathways and normal leptin action. The LEPR isoforms are distributed in almost all peripheral tissues and seem to mediate the transport of LEP. In humans, the effects of LEP can be detected at various sites given that LEPR are found in the brain, heart, placenta, lung, liver, muscle, kidney, pancreas, spleen, thymus, prostate, testes, ovary, small intestine, and colon [46]. Therefore, LEPR locations demonstrate LEP's importance in human molecular processes. The signaling events that follow the binding of LEP to its LEPRs have been studied extensively and characterized at the biochemical and molecular levels in many systems and, more recently, in relation to immune responses [47].

4. Leptin and cancer

LEP is the most studied adipocytokine, particularly in metabolism and obesity-related cancers. It is well established that LEP has pro-tumoral roles; it promotes angiogenesis, proliferation, survival of tumor cells, and inhibits apoptosis [48]. To exercise its role in tumorigenesis, LEP-LEPR signaling and epithelial-mesenchymal transitions (EMTs) play a significant role in tumor initiation, progression, metastasis, and chemoresistance. The function of the leptin axis in cancer is through LEP-LEPR singling. The binding of LEP to LEPR induces the activation of several signaling pathways, such as JAK/STAT3, PI3K/AKT, and MAPK/ERK. Cumulative research demonstrated high levels of LEP and LEPR expression in cancer cells. LEP and LEPR levels are usually missing in epithelial breast tissue but are found in abundance in breast cancer [49]. Other cancers that show high levels of LEP and LEPR include hepatocellular carcinoma [50], lung cancer [51], prostate cancer [52], colorectal cancer [53], melanoma [54], ovarian cancer [55] renal carcinoma [56], and breast cancer (**Figure 2**) [57]. It was also demonstrated that the upregulated level of LEP correlates with clinical and prognostic outcomes in multiple cancer types such as the presence of remote metastasis of breast cancer and the short survival of its patients. The level of LEP expression is influenced by numerous physiological mechanisms, which are noted to be associated with fat mass. One of such mechanisms is the ability of inflammatory cytokines, i.e., TNF-α, interleukin-1 (IL-1), and leukemia inhibitory factor, to induce adipocytes to produce LEP and increase the expression of its mRNA synthesis [58]. Another factor is the genetic variations in the *LEP* gene and/or *LEPR* gene that modulates LEP level [59, 60]. The genetic variations in these genes have been specifically linked to the progression of prostate, breast, gastric, and lung carcinomas [61–63]. Since the proposal of LEP as an EMT inducer a decade ago, research has proven it to be very important in driving the cellular process to aggressive cancer phenotypes. EMT is a complex reprogramming cellular process allowing epithelial cells to acquire mesenchymal characteristics, an important role in the tumor microenvironment (TME). This change enhances migratory and invasive capability and has been demonstrated to be essential in the metastatic spread of several cancer types, including prostate, lung, liver, pancreatic, and breast cancers [64, 65]. EMT programs were also found to stimulate the production of LEP by cancer cells, suggesting a signaling loop in tumor progression. Other important signaling molecules involved in the process

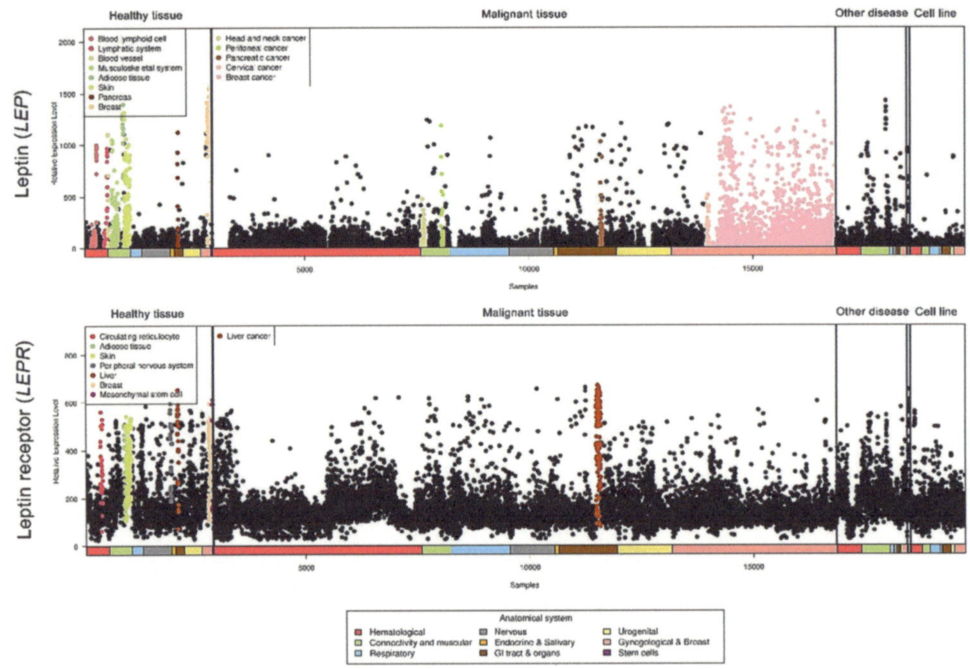

Figure 2.
LEP and LEPR expression in a pancancer panel. From Lin and Hsiao [49].

include integrins, growth factors, and cytokines, such as IL-8, IL-6, and TNF-α, which are often secreted by tumor stroma [66, 67]. Literature has also documented that EMT programs can stimulate the production of proinflammatory factors. Olea-Flores demonstrated the mechanism by which LEP promotes EMT programming, through Src and FAK activations that control the secretion and activation of metalloproteinase-2 (MMP-2) and metalloproteinase-9 (MMP-9). Leptin promotes the expression of EMT-related transcription factors and invasion in a Src and FAK-dependent pathway in MCF10A mammary epithelial cells [68]. In a recent review, Tsung-Chieh and Michael indicated that cancer cells and the tumor microenvironment express LEP and LEPRs and suggested that the potential leptin autocrine/paracrine signaling loop could affect tumor progression [49].

Other studied theories on the involvement of LEP in carcinogenesis were described to be mediated by LEPR activation of PI3K, ERK1/2, and Jak2/Stat3 signaling pathways. These pathways regulate the expression of cancer-related genes, such as cyclin D1, cyclooxygenase-2 (COX-2), vascular endothelial growth factor (VEGF), and potentiate several procarcinogenic processes, including angiogenesis, migration, and mesenchymal transformation [69, 70]. Additionally, *in vitro* studies have documented the antiapoptotic and mitogenic effects of LEP on different cancer cell lines. Zhang and his team have shown that LEP can play the role of being an antiapoptotic by regulating the expression of proteins involved in the apoptotic pathway. They observed that LEP decreases the apoptotic potential of adipose tissue by increasing the Bcl2 and decreasing proapoptotic Bax and CD95 protein expression [71]. More importantly, LEP has been studied as an oncogenic factor due to its proinflammatory and proangiogenic effects.

5. Role of leptin as a proinflammatory factor

The immune system response, acute and chronic inflammation, is called into action when other homeostatic mechanisms are inadequate. Inflammatory mediators play a significant role, adjacent in importance to mutations and epigenetic alterations. In tumor initiation, LEP plays a pleiotropic role in the immune response and can appropriately be considered, both structurally and functionally, as a proinflammatory cytokine. LEP regulates both innate and adaptive immune responses through the modulation of immune cells' survival and proliferation as well as its activity [72–74]. LEP has a modulatory impact on the course of inflammation, affecting the expression of proinflammatory cytokines and their receptors. In the innate immune response, LEP enhances the secretion of TNF-α, a proinflammatory mediator, and interacts with interleukin1beta (IL1β) [75]. IL1β has the ability to increase the levels of cytokines, such as Interleukin 6 (IL6), Interleukin 8 (IL8), and prostaglandin E2 (PGE2), by its mechanism on nitric oxide synthase-2 (NOS2) through the JAK2, PI3K, MAP2K1/MEK1, and MAPK14/p38 signaling pathways [76]. These cytokines also regulate the expression of LEP, creating a signaling loop that supports sustaining a chronic proinflammatory state [77]. In the adaptive immune response, LEP promotes the alteration of memory T-cells immune response toward T helper-1 cells, as well as escalating CD4+CD25– T-cell proliferation and reducing the autophagy process during T-cell receptor (TCR) stimulation by triggering MTOR signaling pathway and upregulating the synthesis of B-cell lymphoma 2 (BCL2) [78]. LEP controls the crosstalk between innate and adaptive immunity by affecting dendritic cell number, maturation, cytokine production, and capacity to induce CD4+ T-cell proliferation [79]. Chronic infectious, immune, and metabolic diseases may lead to LEP resistance, increasing LEP levels and further fueling the inflammatory state. LEP's involvement in the immune and inflammatory response has become increasingly evident and, in turn, is important in cancer.

6. Role of leptin as an angiogenic growth factor

Angiogenesis, a hallmark of cancer, refers to the formation of new blood vessels from preexisting ones. It is a vital process that plays a role in normal physiological as well as pathological processes. Angiogenesis enables tumor growth and metastasis through a multistep progression commencing with endothelial cell migration, proliferation, invasion, and ultimately novel capillary formation. Though the basic steps of angiogenesis are similar in all tissue, it is likely that the vascular network of each organ will be established through tissue-specific key mechanisms. Angiogenesis requires a balance between proangiogenic and antiangiogenic factors; changes in equilibrium can lead to oncogenic angiogenesis.

White adipose tissue is embedded in a dense vascular network and is the most vascularized tissue in the human body. The hypervascularization of the white adipose tissue indicates the presence of an intimate interplay between both the vascular and adipose compartments. The functions of adipose vasculature are summarized in **Table 2**. It has been previously noted that the white adipose tissue regulates the production of various adipocytokines, but it also releases angiogenic factors; therefore, it influences and modulates angiogenesis as well as vascular structure [80–82]. Scientific research has been able to narrow the culprits of angiogenic growth in white

	Adipose vasculature functions
1	Providing nutrients and oxygen essential for the maintenance of adipocyte survival and functions
2	Removing metabolic products from adipose tissue
3	Paracrine regulation of adipocyte functions through the production of various factors and cytokines from vascular cells
4	Transporting adipose-tissue-derived growth factors, adipokines, and cytokines for removal of tissues globally regulating physiological functions via the endocrine mechanism
5	Transporting non-adipose-tissue derived growth factors, cytokines, and hormones for modulating adipocyte functions and growth
6	Alteration of the adipose microenvironment such as hypoxia and acidosis, which control adipocyte function, preadipocyte differentiation, and adipose tissue mass
7	Supplying circulating stem cells from non-adipose tissues to adipose tissues
8	Supplying adipocyte vessel wall stem and precursor cells that can eventually differentiate into mature adipocytes
9	Supplying other cell types such as inflammatory cells that secondarily affect adipocyte function
10	Preparation of adipose niche formation during embryonic development by the vasculature

Table 2.
Adipose vasculature functions in the modulation of adipocyte functions.

adipose tissue to two possibilities: first, in response to signals initiating from neighboring adipocytes that are undergoing proliferation and enlargement; the other possibility is through metabolic signals produced locally or distally. These two possibilities are not mutually exclusive, and probably tissue expansion involves both local signals arising from expanding adipocytes and distant signals reflecting the developmental and metabolic state of the whole organism. It has been acknowledged that adipogenesis, angiogenesis, and vascular remodeling are tightly related and regulated processes. Dysfunction in the regulation of one or more of these processes leads to changes in vessel growth, vascular permeability, remodeling, adipose mass, and function, which will ultimately cause pathological angiogenesis or vascular regression [83].

In white adipose tissue, LEP was found to be an important proangiogenic factor or an angiogenesis inducer [84]. In 1998, Sierra-Honigmann and colleagues produced one of the first studies to demonstrate that leptin-induced cell proliferation, cell survival, and 3D matrix formation of capillary-like tubes mimicking vascular endothelial growth factor (VEGF) 165 [85]. This supported the notion that LEP is an endothelial growth factor. LEP is able to act as a direct factor to induce the angiogenic potential of endothelial cells evident by the presence of LEPR on endothelial cells. Both *in vivo* and *in vitro* studies have demonstrated the activation of endothelial LEPR by LEP, leading to capillary tube formation [86]. The indirect involvement of LEP in angiogenesis has been explored immensely. Garonna *et al.* showed that leptin enhances endothelial cyclooxygenase-2 (COX-2) expression and causes rapid VEGFR2 phosphorylation through the activation of P38 MAPK/AKT/COX-2, which is needed for leptin-stimulated neoangiogenesis [87]. LEP increases the levels and activity of enzymes involved in angiogenesis through metalloproteinase-2 (MMP-2) and MMP-9 activity [82]. Additionally, LEP has been shown to upregulate and act synergistically with the key angiogenic mediators like fibroblast growth factor (FGF)-2, VEGF, and its receptor VEGFR, resulting in stimulation of blood-vessel growth [88]. The VEGF and VEGFR have a special signaling transduction system that plays a significant role in the process of oncogenic angiogenesis. *In vitro* and *in vivo* findings have implicated the role of VEGFR in the facilitation of angiogenic growth and endothelial cell tube development [89]. LEP can upregulate VEGF expression and function, VEGF can, in turn, activate LEP demonstrating the functional interplay between both cytokines. The increase in the presence of both cytokines could generate and amplify a proangiogenic environment. Moreover, crosstalk between LEP and VEGF has been noted in other tissues, such as in cancerous breast tissue; LEP activates HIF-1α and NF-κB to upregulate VEGF [89]. Additionally, LEP is involved in tumor angiogenesis-related signaling pathways such as STAT3/ERK1/2, JAK2/STAT3, MAPK/ERK, PI3K/AKT, p38, p53, MAPK, and Wnt/β-catenin [90]. Less studied are the Akt and Wnt signaling pathways' effect on the proliferation and angiogenic differentiation of endothelial cells, though LEP's involvement was demonstrated [91]. Furthermore, distinct mechanisms, regulated Wnt-responsive GSK-3β and growth factor/Akt responsive GSK-3β, suggest that GSK-3β has a crucial role in the crosstalk between the Akt and Wnt signaling pathways [92]. However, the underlying cellular mechanism remains to be elicited. Of note, tumor angiogenesis is closely associated with the tumor microenvironment and is regulated by a variety of proangiogenic factors and/or angiogenic inhibitors. The genetic and epigenetic alterations of angiogenesis-associated genes might result in angiogenesis dysfunctions and promote tumorigenesis.

Acknowledgements

The author would like to thank Dr. Rayya Alharthi for her support and for editing this chapter.

Author details

Rowyda Nawwaf Al-Harithy
King Abdulaziz University (KAU), Jeddah, Saudi Arabia

*Address all correspondence to: dr.alharithy@gmail.com

References

[1] Kahn CR, Wang G, Lee KY. Altered adipose tissue and adipocyte function in the pathogenesis of metabolic syndrome. The Journal of Clinical Investigation. 2019;**129**(10):3990-4000

[2] Poulos SP, Hausman DB, Hausman G, J. The development and endocrine functions of adipose tissue. Molecular and Cellular Endocrinology. 2010;**323**(1):20-34

[3] Zinngrebe J, Debatin K, Fischer-Posovszky P. Adipocytes in hematopoiesis and acute leukemia: Friends, enemies, or innocent bystanders? Leukemia. 2020;**34**:2305-2316

[4] Schoettl T, Fischer IP, Ussar S. Heterogeneity of adipose tissue in development and metabolic function. The Journal of Experimental Biology. 2018;**7**:221

[5] Bruna B, Brandão BB, Guerra BZ, Mori MA. Shortcuts to a functional adipose tissue: The role of small non-coding RNAs. Redox Biology. 2017;**12**:82-102

[6] Vazquez-Vela ME, Torres N, Tova AR. White adipose tissue as endocrine organ and its role in obesity. Archives of Medical Research. 2008;**39**(8):715-728

[7] Tchoukalova YD, Votruba SB, Tchkonia T, Giorgadze N, Kirkland JL, Jensen MD. Regional differences in cellular mechanisms of adipose tissue gain with overfeeding. Proceedings of the National Academy of Sciences. 2010;**107**(42):18226-18231

[8] Niersmann C, Carstensen-Kirberg M, Maalmi H, Holleczek B, Roden M, Brenner H, et al. Higher circulating omentin is associated with increased risk of primary cardiovascular events in individuals with diabetes. Diabetologia. 2020;**63**:410-418

[9] Juge-Aubry CE, Henrichot E, Meier CA. Adipose tissue a regulator of inflammation. Best Practice & Research. Clinical Endocrinology & Metabolism. 2005;**19**(4):547-566

[10] Ahima RS, Lazar MA. Adipokines and the peripheral and neural control of energy balance. Molecular Endocrinology. 2008;**22**:1023-1031

[11] Zorena K, Jachimowicz-Duda O, Slezak D, Robakowska M, Mrugacz M. Adiokines and obesity. Potential link to metabolic disorders and chronic complications. International Journal of Molecular Sciences. 2020;**21**(10):3570

[12] Cook KS, Min HY, Johnson D, Chaplinsky RJ, Flier JS, Hunt CR, et al. Adipsin: A circulating serine protease homolog secreted by adipose tissue and sciatic nerve. Science. 1993;**237**(4813):402-405

[13] Hotamisligil GS, Shargill NS, Spiegelman BM. Adipose expression of tumor necrosis factor-alpha: Direct role in obesity-linked insulin resistance. Science. 1993;**259**(5091):87-91

[14] Zhang Y, Proenca R, Maffei M, Barone M, Leopold L, Friedman JM. Positional cloning of the mouse obese gene and its human homologue. Nature. 1994;**372**(6505):425-432

[15] Abella V, Scotece M, Conde J, Pino J, Gonzalez-Gay MA, Gómez-Reino JJ, et al. Leptin in the interplay of inflammation, metabolism and immune system disorders. Nature Reviews Rheumatology. 2017;**13**:100-109

[16] Scherer PE, Williams S, Fogliano M, Baldini G, Lodish HF. A novel serum protein similar to C1q, produced exclusively in adipocytes. The Journal of Biological Chemistry. 1995;**270**:26746-26749

[17] Hu E, Liang P, Spiegelman BM. AdipoQ is a novel adipose-specific gene dysregulated in obesity. The Journal of Biological Chemistry. 1996;**271**:10697-10703

[18] Maeda K, Okubo K, Shimomura I, Funahashi T, Matsuzawa Y, Matsubara K. cDNA cloning and expression of a novel adipose specific collagen-like factor, apM1 (AdiPose Most abundant Gene transcript 1). Biochemical and Biophysical Research Communications. 1996;**221**(2):286-289

[19] Ouchi N, Kihara S, Funahashi T, Matsuzawa Y, Walsh K. Obesity, adiponectin and vascular inflammatory disease. Current Opinion in Lipidology. 2003;**14**:561-566

[20] Ouchi N, Walsh K. Adiponectin as an anti-inflammatory factor. Clinica Chimica Acta. 2007;**380**(1-2):24-30

[21] Vega GL, Grundy SM. Metabolic risk susceptibility in men is partially related to adiponectin/leptin ratio. Journal of Obesity. 2013;**2013**:409679

[22] Frühbeck G, Catalán V, Rodríguez A, Gómez-Ambrosi J. Adiponectin-leptin ratio: A promising index to estimate adipose tissue dysfunction. Relation with obesity-associated cardiometabolic risk. Adipocyte. 2018;**7**:57-62

[23] Masuzaki H, Ogawa Y, Sagawa N, Hosoda K, Matsumoto T, et al. Nonadipose tissue production of leptin: Leptin as a novel placenta-derived hormone in humans. Nature Medicine. 1997;**3**(9):1029-1033

[24] Bado A, Levasseur S, Attoub S, Kermorgant S, Laigneau JP, Bortoluzzi MN, et al. The stomach is a source of leptin. Nature. 1998;**394**(6695):790-793

[25] Smith-Kirwin SM, O'Connor DM, Johnston J, de Lancy E, Hassink SG, Funanage VL. Leptin expression in human mammary epithelial cells and breast milk. The Journal of Clinical Endocrinology and Metabolism. 1998;**83**(5):1810-1813

[26] Cinti S, De Matteis R, Pico C, Ceresi E, Obrador A, Maffeis C, et al. Secretory granules of endocrine and chief cells of human stomach mucosa contain leptin. International Journal of Obesity. 2000;**24**(6):789-793

[27] Chan JL, Matarese G, Shetty GK, Raciti P, Kelesidis I, Aufiero D, et al. Differential regulation of metabolic, neuroendocrine, and immune function by leptin in humans. Proceedings of the National Academy of Sciences. 2006;**103**(22):8481-8486

[28] Hausman GJ, Barb CR, Lents CA. Leptin and reproductive function. Biochimie. 2012;**94**(10):2075-2081

[29] Friedman JM. Leptin and the endocrine control of energy balance. Nature Metabolism. 2019;**1**(8):754-764

[30] Licinio J, Negrao AB, Wong ML. Plasma leptin concentrations are highly correlated to emotional states throughout the day. Translational Psychiatry. 2014;**4**(10):e475-e475

[31] Lee SM, Choi HJ, Oh CH, Oh JW, Han JS. Leptin increases TNF-α expression and production through phospholipase D1 in Raw 264.7 cells. PLOS One. 2014;**9**(7):e102373

[32] Stern JH, Rutkowski JM, Scherer PE. Adiponectin, leptin, and fatty acids

in the maintenance of metabolic homeostasis through adipose tissue crosstalk. Cell Metabolism. 2016;**23**(5): 770-784

[33] Kumar R, Mal K, Razaq MK, Magsi M, Memon MK, Memon S, et al. Association of leptin with obesity and insulin resistance. Cureus. 19 Dec 2020;**12**(12):e12178

[34] Dallner OS, Marinis JM, Lu Y-H, Birsoy K, Werner E, Fayzikhodjaeva G, et al. Dysregulation of a long noncoding RNA reduces leptin leading to a leptin-responsive form of obesity. Nature Medicine. 2019;**25**(3):507-516

[35] Salageanu A, Tucureanu C, Lerescu L, Caras I, Pitica R, Gangura G, et al. Serum levels of adipokines resistin and leptin in patients with colon cancer. Journal of Medicine and Life. 2010;**3**:416-420

[36] Riondino S, Roselli M, Palmirotta R, Della-Morte D, Ferroni P, Guadagni F. Obesity and colorectal cancer: Role of adipokines in tumor initiation and progression. World Journal of Gastroenterology. 2014;**20**:5177-5190

[37] Pan H, Deng LL, Cui JQ, Shi L, Yang YC, Luo JH, et al. Association between serum leptin levels and breast cancer risk: An updated systematic review and meta-analysis. Medicine. 2018;**97**:e11345

[38] Andò S, Catalano S. The multifactorial role of leptin in driving the breast cancer microenvironment. Nature Reviews. Endocrinology. 2011;**8**:263-275

[39] Inagaki-Ohara K. Gastric leptin and tumorigenesis: Beyond obesity. International Journal of Molecular Sciences. 2019;**20**(11):2622

[40] Victoria B, Camelia BL. Serum leptin level as a diagnostic and prognostic marker in infectious diseases and sepsis: A comprehensive literature review. Medicine. 2021;**100**(17)

[41] Tartaglia LA, Dembski M, Weng X, Deng N, Culpepper J, Devos R, et al. Identification and expression cloning of a leptin receptor. OB-R. Cell. 1995;**83**:1263-1271

[42] Tartaglia LA. The leptin receptor. The Journal of Biological Chemistry. 1997;**272**:6093-6096

[43] Gorska E, Popko K, Stelmaszczyk-Emmel A, Ciepiela A, Wasik M. Leptin receptors. European Journal of Medical Research. 2010;**15**(2):50

[44] Wauman J, Zabeau L, Tavernier J. The leptin receptor complex: Heavier than expected? Frontiers in Endocrinology. 2017;**8**:30

[45] Peelman F, Zabeau L, Moharanna K, Savvides SN, Tavernier J. Insights into signaling assemblies of leptin receptor. The Journal of Endocrinology. 2014;**223**:T9-T23

[46] Kamel HFM, Nassir AM, Al Refai A. Assessment of expression levels of leptin and leptin receptor as potential biomarkers for risk of prostate cancer development and aggressiveness. Cancer Medicine. 2020;**9**:5687-5696

[47] Kieman K, Maclver NJ. The role of the adipokine leptin in immune cell function in health and disease. Frontiers in Immunology. 2021;**11**:622468

[48] Pham D-V, Park P-H. Tumor metabolic reprogramming by adipokines as a critical driver of obesity-associated cancer progression. International Molecular Scencei. 2021;**22**(3):1444

[49] Lin TC, Hsiao M. Leptin and cancer: Updated functional roles in

carcinogenesis, therapeutic niches, and developments. International Journal of Molecular Sciences. 2021;**22**(6):2870

[50] Ding Y, Cao Y, Wang B, Wang L, Zhang Y, Zhang D, et al. APPL1-mediating leptin signaling contributes to proliferation and migration of cancer cells. PLoS One. 2016;**11**(11):e0166172

[51] Feng H, Liu Q, Zhang N, Zheng L, Sang M, Feng J, et al. Leptin promotes metastasis by inducing an epithelial-mesenchymal transition in A549 lung cancer cells. Oncology Research Featuring Preclinical and Clinical Cancer Therapeutics. 2014;**21**(3):165-171

[52] Price RS, Cavazos DA, De Angel RE, Hursting SD, Degraffenried LA. Obesity-related systemic factors promote an invasive phenotype in prostate cancer cells. Prostate Cancer and Prostatic Diseases. 2012;**15**(2):135-143

[53] Yoon KW, Park SY, Kim JY, Lee SM, Park CH, Cho SB, et al. Leptin-induced adhesion and invasion in colorectal cancer cell lines. Oncology Reports. 2014;**31**(6):2493-2498

[54] Oba J, Wei W, Gershenwald JE, Johnson MM, Wyatt CM, Ellerhorst JA, et al. Elevated serum leptin levels are associated with an increased risk of sentinel lymph node metastasis in cutaneous melanoma. Medicine. 2016;**95**(11):e3073

[55] Wei X, Li Y, Gong C, Ji T, Zhou X, Zhan T, et al. Targeting leptin as a therapeutic strategy against ovarian cancer peritoneal metastasis. Anti-Cancer Agents in Medicinal Chemistry (Formerly Current Medicinal Chemistry-Anti-Cancer Agents). 2017;**17**(8):1093-1101

[56] Campo-Verde-Arbocco F, López-Laur JD, Romeo LR, Giorlando N, Bruna FA, et al. Human renal adipose tissue induces the invasion and progression of renal cell carcinoma. Oncotarget. 2017;**8**(55):94223

[57] Bowers LW, Rossi EL, McDonell SB, Doerstling SS, Khatib SA, Lineberger CG, et al. Leptin signaling mediates obesity-associated CSC enrichment and EMT in preclinical TNBC models. Molecular Cancer Research. 2018;**16**(5):869-879

[58] Palhinha L, Liechocki S, Hottz ED, Aparecida de Pereira J, de Almeida CJ, Moraes-Vieira PM. Leptin induces proadipogenic and proinflammatory signaling in adipocytes. Frontiers in Endocrinology. 2019;**1**(1):15

[59] He J, Xu G. LEP gene variant is associated with prostate cancer but not with colorectal cancer. Tumor Biology. 2013;**34**(5):3131-3136

[60] Dallal C, Garte S, Ragin C, Chen J, Lloyd S, Modugno F, et al. Plasma leptin levels, LEPR Q223R polymorphism and mammographic breast density: A cross-sectional study. The International Journal of Biological Markers. 2013;**28**(2):161-167

[61] Wang LQ, Shen W, Xu L, Chen MB, Gong T, Lu PH, et al. The association between polymorphisms in the leptin receptor gene and risk of breast cancer: A systematic review and pooled analysis. Breast Cancer Research and Treatment. 2012;**136**(1):231-239

[62] Kim EY, Chin HM, Park SM, Jeon HM, Chung WC, Paik CN, et al. Susceptibility of gastric cancer according to leptin and leptin receptor gene polymorphisms in Korea. Journal of the Korean Surgical Society. 2012;**83**(1):7-13

[63] Li Y, Geng J, Wang Y, Lu O, Du Y, Wang W, et al. The role of leptin receptor gene polymorphisms in determining

the susceptibility and prognosis of NSCLC in Chinese patients. Journal of Cancer Research and Clinical Oncology. 2012;**138**(2):311-316

[64] Lin T-C, Huang K-W, Liu C-W, Chang Y-C, Lin W-M, Yang T-Y, et al. Leptin signaling axis specifically associates with clinical prognosis and is multifunctional in regulating cancer progression. Oncotarget. 2018;**9**:17210-17219

[65] Haque I, Ghosh A, Acup S, Banerjee S, Dhar K, Ray A, et al. Leptin-induced ER-α-positive breast cancer cell viability and migration is mediated by suppressing CCN5-signaling via activating JAK/AKT/STAT-pathway. BMC Cancer. 2018;**18**:99

[66] Sullivan NJ, Sasser AK, Axel AE, Vesuna F, Raman V, Ramirez N. Interleukin-6 induces an epithelial-mesenchymal transition phenotype in human breast cancer cells. Oncogene. 2009;**28**(33):2940-2947

[67] Fernando RI, Castillo MD, Litzinger M, Hamilton DH, Palena C. IL-8 signaling plays a critical role in the epithelial-mesenchymal transition of human carcinoma cells. Cancer Research. 2011;**71**(15):5296-5306

[68] Olea-Flores M, Zuñiga-Eulogio M, Tacuba-Saavedra A, Bueno-Salgado M, Sánchez-Carvajal A, Vargas-Santiago Y, et al. Leptin promotes expression of EMT-related transcription factors and invasion in a Src and FAK-dependent pathway in MCF10A mammary epithelial cells. Cells. 2019;**8**(10):1133

[69] Lim SC. Role of COX-2, VEGF and cyclin D1 in mammary infiltrating duct carcinoma. Oncology Reports. 2003;**10**(5):1241-1249

[70] Jimenez-Cortegana C, Lopez-Saavedra A, Sanchez-Jimenez F, Perez-Perez A, Castineiras J, Virizuela-Echaburu JA, et al. Leptin, both bad and good actor in cancer. Biomolecules. 2021;**11**(6):913

[71] Zange Y, Somers VK, Dong Y, Singh P. Abstract 604: Anti-apoptotic role of leptin in adipose tissue. Arteriosclerosis, Thrombosis, and Vascular Biology. 2019;**38**(1):604

[72] Procaccini C, Lourenco EV, Matarese G, Cava AL. Leptin signaling: A key pathway in immune responses. Current Signal Transduction Therapy. 2009;**4**(1):22-30

[73] La Cava A. Leptin in inflammation and autoimmunity. Cytokine. 2017;**98**:51-58

[74] Song J, Deng T. Corrigendum: The adipocyte and adaptive immunity. Frontiers in Immunology. 2021;**12**

[75] Pérez-Pérez A, Sánchez-Jiménez F, Vilariño-García T, Sánchez-Margalet V. Role of leptin in inflammation and vice versa. International Journal of Molecular Science. 2020;**21**(16):5587

[76] Agrawal S, Gollapudi S, Su H, Gupta S. Leptin activates human Bcells to secrete TNF-α, IL-6, and IL-10 via JAK_2/$STAT_3$ and P^{38}MARK/ERK1/2 signaling pathway. Journal of Clinical Immunology. 2011;**31**(3):472-478

[77] Finck BN, Johnson RW. Tumor necrosis factor (TNF)-α induces leptin production through the p55 TNF receptor. American Journal of Physiology. Regulatory, Integrative and Comparative Physiology. 2000;**278**:R537-R543

[78] Hardwick JM, Soane L. Multiple functions of BCL-2 family proteins. Cold Spring Harbor Perspectives in Biology. 2013;**5**(2):a008722

[79] Zou Z, Tao T, Li H, Zhu X. mTOR signaling pathway and mTOR inhibitors in cancer: Progress and challenges. Cell & Bioscience. 2020;**10**:31

[80] Kim SY, Lim JH, Choi SW, Kim M, Kim ST, Kim MS, et al. Preferential effects of leptin on CD4 T cells in central and peripheral immune system are critically linked to the expression of leptin receptor. Biochemical and Biophysical Research Communications. 2010;**394**(4):562-568

[81] Herold J, Kalucka J. Angiogenesis in adipose tissue: The interplay between adipose and endothelial cells. Frontiers in Physiology. 2021;**11**:624903

[82] Park HY, Kwon HM, Lim HJ, Hong BK, Lee JY, Park BE, et al. Potential role of leptin in angiogenesis: Leptin induces endothelial cell proliferation and expression of matrix metalloproteinases in vivo and in vitro. Experimental & Molecular Medicine. 2001;**33**(2):95-102

[83] Nagy JA, Benjamin L, Zeng H, Dvorak AM, Dvorak HF. Vascular permeability, vascular hyperpermeability and angiogenesis. Angiogenesis. 2008;**11**(2):109-119

[84] Gonzalez-Perez RR, Lanier V, Newman G. Leptin's pro-angiogenic signature in breast cancer. Cancers. 2013;**5**(3):1140-1162

[85] Sierra-Honigmann MR, Nath AK, Murakami C, García-Cardeña G, Papapetropoulos A, Sessa WC, et al. Biological action of leptin as an angiogenic factor. Science. 1998;**281**:1683-1686

[86] Samad N, R., T. Role of leptin in cancer-a systematic review. Biomedical Journal of Scientific & Technical Research. 2019;**18**(1):13226-13235

[87] Garonna E, Botham KM, Birdsey GM, Randi AM, Gonzalex-Perez RR, Wheeler-Jones CPD. Vascular endothelial growth factor receptor-2 couples cyclo-oxygenase-2 with pro-angiogenic actions of leptin on human endothelial cells. PLoS One. 2011;**6**(4):e18823

[88] Cao R, Brakenhielm E, Wahlestedt C, Thyberg J, Cao Y. Leptin induces vascular permeability and synergistically stimulates angiogenesis with FGF-2 and VEGF. Proceedings of the National Academy of Sciences. 2001;**98**(11):6390-6395

[89] Guo S, Colbert LS, Fuller M, Zhang Y, Gonzalez-Perez RR. Vascular endothelial growth factor receptor-2 in breast cancer. Biochimica et Biophysica Acta. 2010;**1806**:108-121

[90] Zhou W, Guo S, Gonzalez-Perez RR. Leptin pro-angiogenic signature in breast cancer is linked to IL-1 signalling. British Journal of Cancer. 2011;**104**:128-137

[91] Pua LJW, Mai CW, Chung FFL, Khoo ASB, Leong CO, Lim WM, et al. Functional roles of JNK and p38 MAPK signaling in nasopharyngeal carcinoma. International Journal of Molecular Sciences. 2022;**23**(3):1108

[92] Liang X, Wang S, Wang X, Zhang L, Zha H, Zhang L. Leptin promotes the growth of breast cancer by upregulating the Wnt/β-catenin pathway. Experimental and Therapeutic Medicine. 2018;**16**(2):767-771

Chapter 8

Extracellular Matrix in Tumor Angiogenesis

Gvantsa Kharaishvili

Abstract

Extracellular matrix (ECM) is a complex three-dimensional network that provides structure, strength, and contextual information for cellular growth, communication, differentiation, survival, adhesion, and migration. ECM basic proteins resist compressive forces and/or allow rapid diffusion, others strengthen the matrix, and give resilience or modulate cell-matrix interactions. ECM undergoes turnover and remodeling physiologically and during inflammation, wound repair and tumor invasion. Remodeling of the ECM is an integral component of the angiogenic process and depends on the composition of matrix molecules, soluble pro-angiogenic and anti-angiogenic factors, and their spatial regulation. This review will focus on the myriad roles of those molecules and will emphasize their involvement in critical points of angiogenesis.

Keywords: extracellular matrix, tumor microenvironment, angiogenesis, pro-angiogenic, anti-angiogenic

1. Introduction

"Tumor progression is defined by irreversible change in the tumor characteristics reflecting the sequential appearance of a genetically altered subpopulation of cells with the new characteristics" [1]. The term, "tumor progression" is used to describe phenotypic changes in the preexisting neoplastic lesion. It is a coincidence of complex events characterized by morphological, molecular, and functional changes in tumor cells and their environment and encompasses a wide scale of mechanisms [2]. It is in part recognized as a product of evolving crosstalk between different cell types within the tumor and its surrounding supportive tissue or tumor stroma [3]. Invasive tumor cells interact with their microenvironment in a bidirectional manner and remodel it into a supportive context for tumor growth and progression. The composition of the tumor microenvironment varies between tumor types, but hallmark features include cellular components such as immune cells (T-cells, B-cells, NK-cells, macrophages, neutrophils, dendritic cells), stromal cells, blood vessels, cancer-associated fibroblasts, adipocytes, stellate cells, and noncellular components such as extracellular matrix (ECM) and exosomes [4].

2. Extracellular matrix: its composition and molecular profile

Extracellular matrix (ECM) is a noncellular, proteinaceous component of the stroma. It is a complex three-dimensional network of macromolecules. The ECM provides architectural structure, strength, and contextual information for cellular growth, adhesion, communication, differentiation, migration, and survival. Molecules that provide ECM structure are: glycosaminoglycans and proteoglycans (form a hydrated gel-like substance, resist compressive forces, and allow rapid diffusion) and fibrous proteins and collagens (strengthens the matrix and give resilience). They represent insoluble factors of the matrix [5]. Structural molecules are synthesized mainly by fibroblasts but also by other cells of connective tissue. ECM molecules named, "matricellular proteins" (e.g. thrombospondin-1 and -2, SPARC, tenascin-C, and osteopontin) do not function as structural elements but modulate cell-matrix interactions and cell functions [6]. ECM is in a dynamic state and undergoes turnover and remodeling in conjunction with signals and is enhanced during inflammation, wound repair, and tumor invasion. However, ECM can limit initiation of tumor at an early stage of its development, later, ECM stimulates tumor growth and progression and enhances its aggressiveness. Key enzymes which remodel ECM are matrix metalloproteinases (MMPs) and urokinase-type plasminogen activators (uPAs). They degrade components of the basement membrane as well as proteins and proteoglycans of connective tissue and liberate latent growth factors from their storage sites in the extracellular matrix. Factors that are activated in this fashion are, for example, fibroblast growth factors (FGFs), hepatocyte growth factor (HGF), and transforming growth factors (TGFs) [7]. Tumor growth-induced solid stress, matrix stiffness, increased interstitial fluid pressure, hypoxia and altered tumor pH have been established as a result of tumor growth and on the other hand, neoangiogenesis-supporting conditions. As structural and metabolic alterations of ECM can lead to the development or progression of disease, its molecules can serve as important targets for pharmacotherapy.

2.1 Collagens

Collagen represents 30% of dry weight in the human body and is the most abundant protein synthesized by fibroblasts and by several other cell types distinct by their molecular profile, morphology, distribution function, and involvement in pathologies [8]. Collagens play structural roles and contribute to mechanical properties, organization, and configuration of tissues. Some collagens have a restricted tissue distribution and hence specific biological functions [9]. Collagens are trimeric molecules composed of three polypeptide α chains, which contain the sequence repeat that allows the formation of a triple helix. Besides triple-helical domains, collagens contain non-triple-helical domains, used as building blocks by other extracellular matrix proteins. At present, 28 types of collagens are classified as fibrillar collagens, unconventional collagens including collagen VII, network-forming collagens (VI, VIII, and X), fibril-associated collagens with interrupted triple helix (IX, XII, XIV, XVI, and XIX), basement membrane collagens, transmembrane collagens, and multiplexins [10, 11]. Type I, II, III, V, XI, XXIV, and XXVII collagens belong to the classical fibrillar collagens [12]. Fibrillar collagens can assemble into supramolecular aggregates. Type I collagen is major collagen of tendons, ligaments, skin, cornea, and other connective tissues representing 90% of the total collagen in humans. It is mostly a part of the compound containing either type III collagen seen in skin and reticular fibers [13] or type V collagen found in bone [14]. The biomechanical properties of these compounds (e.g., torsional stability and stiffness or tensile strength) establish the stability and integrity of these tissues [15]. Bourgot and colleagues describe the evolution of fibrillar collagen organization during tumor progression where tumor-derived paracrine signals promote a desmoplasic reaction characterized by the activation of the resident fibroblasts into cancer-associated fibroblasts (CAFs) with enhanced secretory activity, reorganization of the collagen fibers (their cross-linking), augmenting the stiffness of the stroma. Tumor adjacent collagen fibers that promote invasive cancer cell migration can be organized parallel (Tumor Associated Collagen Signature—TACS-2) or perpendicular to the tumor border (TACS-3) [16]. Collagen fibers employ guidance signals for endothelial cell migration during regenerative angiogenesis. Inhibition of collagen cross-linking results in a 70% shorter regeneration area with 50% reduced vessel growth and disintegrated collagen fibers. The disrupted collagen scaffold impedes endothelial cell migration and induces the formation of abnormal angioma-like blood vessels [16]. Type I collagen, potently stimulates angiogenesis in vitro and in vivo [17]. Crucial to its angiogenic activity appears to be ligation and possibly clustering of endothelial cell surface α1β1/α2β1 integrin receptors by the GFPGER (502–507) sequence of the collagen fibril. Authors describe here genetically engineered "angiogenic superpolymers", containing type I collagen, fibrillar collagens and collagen mimetics, possibilities of their modifications to display ideal angiogenic properties, and prove their usefulness for tissue engineering and human medicine [17].

The vascular basement membrane represents an insoluble structural component of the wall of newly formed capillaries and undergoes several changes during tumor-induced angiogenesis. Initially, the membrane is degraded and disassembled by proteolytic activity of matrix metalloproteinases, mainly MMP2 and 9, but is finally after complex molecular crosstalk by regulation mainly via VEGF signaling, is reorganized to a native state around a newly formed capillary. Such vascular matrix changes during angiogenesis are associated with the expression of matrix proteins that can interact with vascular endothelium and provide endogenous angiogenic and anti-angiogenic signals. Basement membrane molecules play a role also in the process of the relapse of pathological angiogenesis [18]. Rapid relapse of tumor angiogenesis is hypothesized to be facilitated by the empty basement membrane sleeves (ebms) of previously regressed vessels, which are postulated to serve as scaffolding for endothelial cells during new angiogenic sprouting, following cessation of antiangiogenic treatment [19]. Type IV collagen is found in solid and soluble states in ECM, it is composed of three α(IV) chains [20]. The a1 and a2 isoforms are ubiquitously present in human basement membranes. Type IV collagen promotes cell adhesion, migration, differentiation, growth [21], and regulates endothelial cell proliferation and behavior during the critical steps of the angiogenic process. Studies have shown that the function of type IV collagen in the elongation and stabilization of microvessels was dose-dependent with low concentrations of type IV collagen promoting elongation, and high concentrations stabilizing them. Anti-angiogenic properties were associated with inhibitors of collagen metabolism and basement membrane collagen synthesis and deposition were crucial for blood vessel formation and survival [18]. There are six known bioactive peptides generated from collagen type IV [22]. These peptides are fragments of non-collagenous domains from the α1 (arresten), α2 (canstatin), α3 (tumstatin), α4 (tetrastatin), α5 (pentastatin), and α6 chains (hexastatin). Arresten, is an inhibitor of angiogenesis in squamous cell carcinoma, binding with α1β1 integrin in endothelial cells [22–24]. Carcinoma cells showing overexpression of arresten changed to an endothelial phenotype, suggesting inhibition of migrating carcinoma cells by inducing mesenchymal to endothelial (MET) transition [24]. Role of arresten is demonstrated in modulating the function of capillary endothelial cells and blood vessel formation using in vitro and in vivo models of angiogenesis and tumor growth [25]. Recently, the NC1 domain of the α2 chain of type IV collagen (canstatin) was also identified as an angiogenesis inhibitor. In the study by [25], Canstatin was first identified as vasculogenic mimicry (VM) inhibitor. Vasculogenic mimicry is a neovascularization phenomenon that was first reported in melanoma models. Distinct from classical tumor angiogenesis, VM provides a blood supply for tumor cells independent of endothelial cells and formed by deregulated tumor cells. VM is established in lung cancer [26], hepatocellular carcinoma [27], and glioma [28] and is associated with poor prognosis in cancer patients [29]. Vautrin-Glabik demonstrated that 13 amino acid sequence of tetrastatin decreases VEGF-induced-angiogenesis in vivo using the Matrigel plug model and decreases Human Umbilical Vein Endothelial Cells (HUVEC) migration and pseudotube formation in vitro [30]. Oskimaki et al. recently developed a bioinformatics-based approach to predict over 100 novel endogenous anti-angiogenic peptides [31]. An important peptides determined were tetrastatins, pentastatins, and hexastatins that were validated in vitro in cell proliferation and migration assays on HUVECs [32]. Using pentastatin-1 to an angioreactor-based directed in vivo angiogenesis assay (DIVAA), and in vivo NCI-H82 SCLC xenograft model strong potential for pentastatin-1 as a therapeutic agent for lung cancer was demonstrated [30].

2.2 Elastin

Elastin provides elasticity to the ECM. Elastin is roughly 1000 times more flexible than collagens. It is produced as tropoelastin, a 72 kDa precursor protein by fibroblasts, smooth muscle cells, chondrocytes, or endothelial cell and is secreted from the cell to the extracellular space, where it crosslinks with other elastin molecules. Elastin is the primary ECM protein present in arteries where it composes ~50% of their dry weight [33]. During aging, continuous mechanical stress and an increase in elastase activity contribute to the fragmentation of elastic fibers resulting in the release of elastin-derived peptides (EDPs) [34]. EDPs are matrikines—matrix fragments having the ability to regulate cell physiology and display a wide range of biological activities in a number of normal and transformed cells [35]. For example, they potentiate the migration and matrix invasion of tumor cells, stimulate the migration and proliferation of monocytes and skin fibroblasts and up-regulate MMP expression by fibroblasts inducing a remodeling program for melanoma invasion. Additionally, they are pro-angiogenic, chemotactic for inflammatory cells and promote elastase release [36]. Robinet and colleagues showed that elastin-derived peptides enhanced angiogenesis in the chick chorio-allantoic membrane in vivo, augmented pseudotube formation from human vascular and microvascular endothelial cells in the matrigel and promoted cell migration in wound healing assay [37].

2.3 Glycosaminoglycans

Glycosaminoglycans (GAGs) were primarily known as "space fillers" in the ECM, but later appeared as active signaling molecules in cell fate regulation via cytokine production, leukocyte recruitment, or inflammatory response [38]. GAGs are linear polysaccharides with two basic saccharide molecules that vary according to epimerization, sulfation, and deacetylation. Their specificity and functionality depend on the order of the carbohydrate chain and the other chemical modifications [38]. Hyaluronan is the simplest GAG since it is non-sulfated, does not undergo epimerization, and does not use typical covalent bonds for linking to proteins. Other GAGs—chondroitin sulfate, dermatan sulfate, keratan sulfate, and heparan sulfate usually use covalent bonds for attachment to proteins in proteoglycan molecules. Chondroitin and heparan sulfate are further remodeled by sulfation [33, 39]. Hyaluronan is synthesized at the plasma membrane by transmembrane enzymes of the HA synthase family (HAS1–3) [40, 41]. Chain length is dependent on polymerizing enzyme type, for example, HAS1 and HAS2 produce high molecular weight (~2000 kDa) HA and HAS3 produce lower molecular weight (100–1000 kDa) HA. After synthesis via HASes, extracellular HA can be rapidly altered due to its impressive turnover rate via a variety of hyaluronidases (mainly HYAL1 and 2) [40]. Despite the relative simplicity of its molecule, HA regulates a variety of cellular functions including wound repair, inflammation, cell migration, and angiogenesis [41, 42], and recently emerged as a key player in regulating the tumorigenic and inflammatory milieu [43]. Interestingly, its physiological sequel is largely related to the size of the molecule, for example, full-length HA mainly demonstrates anti-inflammatory property whereas its smaller fragments exert pro-inflammatory and pro-angiogenic features [40]. In cancer and other pathologic states, HA fragments are abundantly deposited in the extracellular environment that, in one hand, is a result of increased synthesis of HA via HASes and on the other hand—accelerated degradation via hyaluronidases, reactive oxygen species, and mechanical forces [44] creating a microenvironment supporting angiogenesis and inflammation [41, 45, 46]. Several evidence suggests that aberrant levels of HAS2 promote breast cancer growth, differentiation, lymph node involvement, and worse patient survival [47, 48]. HAS2 knockdown inhibited breast cancer growth and attenuated HA expression. Similarly, HAS2 has a regulatory effect on tumorigenicity and metastasis of prostate, colon, and ovarian tumors through excessive HA synthesis [49, 50]. Recently, Chen and colleagues [40] suggested a novel mechanism of angiogenesis regulation via autophagic degradation of HAS2 in endothelial cells. In [51], colleagues showed that the C-terminal module of perlecan, endorepellin, blocks VEGFR2 kinase activity, thereby evoking a strong pro-autophagic and anti-angiogenic response in vascular endothelial cells both ex vivo and in vivo. Bix and colleagues [52] have also shown that systemic delivery of recombinant endorepellin inhibits tumor growth and angiogenesis and increases tumor hypoxia in squamous and Lewis lung carcinoma xenograft models. Recently, HAS2 was degraded in vascular endothelial cells via autophagy evoked by nutrient deprivation, mTOR inhibition, or pro-autophagic proteoglycan fragments endorepellin and endostatin [40]. Autophagic degradation of HAS2 suppressed extracellular hyaluronan and inhibited ex vivo angiogenesis showed in aortic ring assay where they quantified the extent of active sprouting issued from the aortic rings and measured the radial distance of the newly-formed vessels where they found a significant reduction in angiogenesis [40]. The antiangiogenic activity of the role of endostatin and tumstatin was also emphasized, where tumor suppressor protein p53 prevented an incipient tumor from switching to the angiogenic phenotype mediated in part by endostatin and tumstatin [53].

The role of tumor-associated macrophages in angiogenesis is documented in [54]. TAMs induce tumor vascularization by releasing several factors, including VEGF which is the main angiogenic factor [55]. Monocytes (Mo) and monocyte-derived macrophages (MØ) can bind HA which induces intracellular signals [56, 57], however, the anti-tumor or pro-tumor role, is dependent on the size of HA in colorectal and breast carcinomas. As it is shown in [55] tumor necrosis factor (TNF)-stimulated gene 6 (TSG-6) was downregulated in Mo/MØ by high molecular weight hyaluronan, modulating their angiogenic behavior in breast carcinoma milieu, but not in colorectal carcinoma [55].

2.4 Proteoglycans

Next to collagens, proteoglycans (PGs) constitute a major class of extracellular matrix/cell surface components known to be involved in primary physiological and pathological phenomena; and due to the altered transcription/translation patterns that these PGs exhibit, they have been identified as potential diagnostic/prognostic and therapeutic targets in diverse disease states [58]. Based upon its direct involvement in cell-cell and cell-ECM interactions, this gene family has been strongly implicated in the regulation of cell movement. Assignment of diverse roles of PGs in promoting, or inhibiting, cell movement seems to be dictated by the biological system [58]. The proteoglycan superfamily now contains more than 30 molecules. They sustain the transparency of the cornea, the elasticity of blood vessels, the tensile strength of the skin, tendon, or cartilage, as well as compressive forces of the mineralized matrix of bones. PGs can alter the biology of growth factors and cytokines [59]. The basic proteoglycan unit consists of a "core protein" with one or more covalently attached glycosaminoglycan chain(s). Proteoglycans can be categorized depending upon the nature of their glycosaminoglycan chains and/or by size (kDa). Four major classes of PGs exist: (i) chondroitin sulfate/dermatan sulfate PGs (decorin, biglycan, versican); heparan sulfate/ chondroitin sulfate PGs (testican, perlecan); (ii) chondroitin sulfate (neurocan, aggrecan); (iii) keratan sulfate (fibromodulin, lumican). Among them, decorin, biglycan, testican, fibromodulin, lumican are small proteoglycans, and versican, perlecan, neurocan, and aggrecan are large proteoglycans. The small leucine-rich repeat proteoglycans (SLRPs) form a group of molecules on the basis of their relatively small protein core (36–42 kDa) [60, 61]. Some of these gene products are not classical proteoglycans. Despite being structural proteins, SLRPs constitute a network of signal regulation: being mostly extracellular, they are upstream of multiple intracellular signaling cascades. They affect intracellular phosphorylation and modulate pathways, including those driven by bone morphogenetic protein/transforming growth factor β superfamily members, receptor tyrosine kinases such as ErbB, and the insulin-like growth factor I receptor, and Toll-like receptors.

Decorin was originally discovered as a collagen-binding protein necessary for fibrillogenesis [62, 63], hence related eponym of decorin [64]. Soluble decorin is a high-affinity antagonistic ligand for several key receptor tyrosine kinases resulting in protracted oncostasis and angiostasis [65]. Recently, decorin has emerged as a soluble pro-autophagic cue by initiating endothelial cell autophagy through activation of AMPK, an energy sensor kinase, and evoking tumor cell mitophagy as the mechanistic basis for the oncostatic effects [66]. Decorin, due to its role as a tumor repressor and anti-angiogenic factor was designated as "a guardian from the matrix" [67]. According to the review, decorin suppresses tumor growth and angiogenesis via EGFR and Met where decorin monomer binds a narrow region of an epitope that in part overlaps with the agonist binding site [68]. This binding further augments receptor dimerization, the consequence of which is rapid phosphorylation of the intracellular tails [69]. This event further recruits and activates downstream effectors, e.g. provides caveosome-mediated internalization of the decorin/receptor complex, and eventual degradation in lysosomes [70, 71]. The latter causes a protracted cessation of intracellular receptor signaling. As a major consequence of inhibiting Met, two potent oncogenes, β-catenin, and Myc, are targeted for sustained degradation via the 26S proteasome [72]. Decorin suppresses β-catenin signaling in a non-canonical fashion and the latter is targeted for degradation in a manner consistent with direct phosphorylation of β-catenin by an RTK, such as Met [73–75]. Wnt/β-catenin signaling activation and its member molecule mutations are well established in colorectal cancer and different epithelial tumor sprouting and nonsprouting angiogenesis. Wnt agonists (e.g., B cell Lymphoma 9 protein (BCL9) is the angiogenesis promoting, where antagonists such as the DKK-4 (also called the Dickkopf Wnt signaling pathway inhibitor 4), in particular, conditioned media from DKK-4 expressing cells promoted the migrative abilities of CRC and formation of capillary-like tubules of human primary microvascular endothelial cells [76].

Versican is a large chondroitin sulfate proteoglycan that forms aggregates with hyaluronan which connects it to the cell surface via hyaluronan receptors such as CD44 [77, 78]. Versican is implicated in many biological processes involving vasculature, such as atherosclerosis and vasculitis [79, 80]. There are five known versican splice isoforms; V0–V4 [81]. Each isoform except V3 has a glycosaminoglycan (GAG) domain with covalently attached chondroitin sulfate (CS) chains. Versican is highly expressed in the early stages of development but becomes downregulated after tissue maturation [82], interestingly, it is reexpressed during wound repair, arteriopathies, pulmonary fibrosis, or tumor formation [83]. Versican is anti-adhesive since it is a poor cell attachment and migration substrate and is excluded from focal adhesions [77, 84, 85]. Several clinical studies have suggested that high versican expression is a poor prognostic factor in gastric, pancreatic, head and neck squamous, or mammary cancers [77]. Increased versican immunostaining has been detected during tumor blood vessel formation [86]. Versican V2 isoform is the major type expressed in brain tissues, and brain tumors are greatly enriched in vascularization, therefore, authors hypothesized that the V2 isoform may play a role in angiogenesis in brain tumors. They injected U87 glioblastoma cells stably transfected with a versican V2 expression construct or a control vector into nude mice and showed that the tumors formed by the V2-transfected cells were visibly enriched in vascularisation, whereas the tumors formed by the vector-transfected cells did not exhibit this phenotype [86]. Furthermore, V2 expression facilitated endothelial-tumor cell interaction observed in tube-like structure formation in matrigel [82]. Koyama and colleagues demonstrated that basic fibroblast growth factor-induced neovascularization was elevated in the presence of either hyaluronan oligosaccharides or a hyaluronan aggregate containing versican, using the Matrigel plug assay. Administration of hyaluronan-versican aggregates, but not native hyaluronan alone, promoted stromal cell recruitment with the infiltration of endothelial cells, suggesting that hyaluronan overproduction accelerates tumor angiogenesis through stromal reaction, notably in the presence of versican [87]. Versican localized preferentially to the vicinity of tumor vasculature and macrophages in the tumor. However, the extracellular protease ADAMTS-generated versican fragment is uniquely localized to vascular endothelium. Members of the family of A disintegrin-like and metalloproteinase with thrombospondin type 1 motifs (ADAMTS) are involved in versican proteolysis and tumor progression [88, 89]. ADAMTS1 was first shown to display anti-angiogenic properties [90]. Later, it's angiostatic (antiangiogenic) and tumor-suppressive properties have also been shown in model systems [91, 92], but controversial results about its relevance to metastasis and tumor growth have also gained attention [93]. ADAMTS family of secreted zinc-dependent metalloproteinases comprises at least 19 genetically distinct members in humans [94]. The expression of the majority of ADAMTS subtypes is associated with pre- and postnatal growth and onset and progression of cancer [95]. ADAMTS subtypes have been sub-classified as aggrecanases because of their ability to cleave large chondroitin sulfate. Despite their structural similarity to other matrix metalloproteinases, ADAMTS have a narrow substrate specificity. This feature could serve as an advantage for ADAMTS inhibitors in the treatment of cancer [95].

Asporin, also known as periodontal ligament-associated protein 1 (PLAP1) was identified in 2001 [96, 97]. Asporin mRNA was expressed primarily in the skeleton (perichondrium/periosteum of cartilage/bone) and other specialized connective tissues. Asporin blocks chondrogenesis and inhibits TGF-β1-induced expression of matrix genes and the resulting chondrocyte phenotypes [98]. Knockdown of asporin increases the expression of cartilage marker genes and TGF-β1; in turn, TGF-β1 stimulates asporin expression in articular cartilage cells, suggesting that asporin and TGF-β1 form a regulatory feedback loop. Asporin, like decorin, can bind collagen at the same site, but in contrast to decorin and biglycan, it drives collagen biomineralization [99]. Our laboratory has identified asporin as a novel cancer-related protein in invasive breast cancer [100]. Later, asporin was reported as an important player in tumor microenvironment [101] and experimentally proved that MDA-MB-231 and BT-549 cells invaded faster through collagen matrix which was prepared with the recombinant asporin. This finding was explained to be related to a less dense matrix due to the inhibition of collagen fibrillogenesis by asporin [102]. Recently, asporin was specifically reported in pancreas and prostate cancer by two additional groups [103, 104]. The direct role of asporin in angiogenesis/angiostasis is not been studied yet, however, a search of the Gene Expression Omnibus, revealed high levels of ASPN expression in white adipose-derived (WAT) CD34+ cells that are a very rich reservoir of CD45− CD34+ populations with endothelial differentiation potential/significantly increased levels of angiogenesis-related genes [101]. The multifaceted role of asporin was recently reviewed also in [105] where its emerging role in proliferation, migration, invasion, and angiogenesis through TGF-β, EGFR, and CD44 pathways was described [105].

2.5 Laminin

Laminins are major noncollagenous constituents of the basement membrane. The fragmentation or absence of BM structures seen in malignant tumors is due to active proteolytic degradation, decreased synthesis of BM components, and/or remodeling by the tumor cells [106]. There are 5α, 4β, and 6γ chains of laminin molecule [33]. It has three short and one long arm arranged in a cross-like structure. The α chains have a larger G domain at the C-termini, which is composed of 3 LG domains (LG1-LG3) connected by a binding region to other LG4 and 5 domains. Integrins bind to LG1–3. Heparan sulfate has been shown to bind to LG4 of the α1 chain. Certain laminin isoforms are predominant in vascular basement membranes and may be critical in maintaining the proper development as well as stability of the mature vessel [107]. LN-1 provoked angiogenesis in the chicken chorioallantoic membrane in the same manner as FGF-2, and vessel development in embryoid bodies was further enhanced in a synergistic mode by FGF-2 and LN-1. The latter significantly enhanced the differentiation of endothelial cells in a 3D collagen environment, either in the absence or presence of FGF-2 [108]. In tumors, as in normal tissues, the blood vessels express laminin α4, α5, β1, and γ1 chains, suggesting the presence of laminin-8 and -10, synthesized by VECs. Laminin-10 is more adhesive and migration promoting [109]. Microvessels are expected to express additional laminins α2, α3, and β2 [107]. The cellular origin of the laminin chains in the vessel should be carefully examined, since pericytes are also able to synthesize several laminins [110]. Lugassy and colleagues [111] in their work studied qualitative aspects of tumor cells and vasculature in melanoma and focused on the pericellular matrix. They demonstrated the angio-tumoral complex in which the tumor cell and endothelium are in direct contact via an amorphous matrix. This amorphous matrix lacks an organized lamina and contains predominantly laminin with noticeably less collagen type IV. Interestingly, this was absent in naevi. Authors regarded the laminin found in this amorphous matrix as "free" laminin, is distinct from laminin integrated into an organized lamina, and showed free laminin role in promoting the migration of melanoma cells in contact with vessels and suggested that this angio-tumoral complex represents a marker for metastasis [112]. During intravasation, tumor cells penetrate BM rich in laminin-8 and 10. When in circulation, large tumor cells and cell aggregates are often covered with platelets, that contain and, following stimulation, secrete laminin-8 and other laminin isoforms [113]. Tumor cell extravasation again requires penetration of the vascular BM to generate secondary tumors [107]. Interaction of tumor cells with endothelial cells and the basement membrane seems organ-specific, time and tumor type-dependent in the ultrastructural study on lung, liver, brain, kidney, and adrenal tissues. Study shows that endothelial cells of the lungs and liver can play a much more active role in the process of extravasation [114]. Laminin α3B chain normally expressed in vascular and epithelial basement membranes, was downregulated in skin cancers [115]. Notably, endothelial cell behavior during tumor progression is largely dependent on complex interactions between laminin molecules with integrins (please see also below).

2.6 Fibronectin

Fibronectin is a dimer with a molecular weight of ~270 kDa. There are two fibronectin forms, soluble plasma fibronectin (p-fibronectin), produced by hepatocytes and cellular fibronectin (c-fibronectin) produced in tissues where it is further deposited as a component of the fibrillar matrix. Many of the functions of fibronectin depend on the 3-dimensional structure of the protein and its assembly into a functional fibrillar matrix [116]. In ECM, fibronectin binds collagen, heparin, other fibronectin proteins, and cell surface integrins. Fibronectin binds integrins through the tripeptide motif of arginine, glycine, and aspartic acid (RGD)2,3, α5β1 integrin plays here a major role. Studies to elucidate the mechanisms of fibronectin fibrillogenesis in endothelial cells have revealed a determinant role for integrin beta subunit adaptor (ILK) in this process [117]. Example of how transient c-fibronectin expression participates in a "pro-angiogenic switch" comes from studies on vascular patterning in the developing retinal vasculature [118, 119]. During this process, blood vessels use the existing astrocyte network as a template, and fibronectin is the principal component of the astrocyte-derived extracellular scaffold. Bazigou et al. [120] showed that interaction between integrin α9 and fibronectin containing the EDA domain is required for fibronectin matrix assembly during lymphatic valve morphogenesis [120]. Targeted deletion of α4 in lymphatic vessels or pharmacological inhibition of α4β1 compromise growth factor- and tumor-induced lymphangiogenesis and suppressed metastatic spread in vivo. α4β1 and c-fibronectin were suggested as markers of proliferative lymphatic endothelium in malignant tumors [121].

Fibronectin is a Wnt target gene and lung vascularization and branching morphogenesis are dependent on Wnt and fibronectin signaling [122]. However, fibronectin level is weak in morphogenesis and quiescent vasculature and highly upregulated together with tenascin-C following vessel injury. Tenascin-C expression is also highly associated with angiogenesis in a wide range of disease states, including diabetes, aortic aneurysm, artherosclerosis, ulcerative colitis, inflammatory bowel disease, Crohn's disease, vasculitis, and cancer [122]. Both proteins were localized in the vessel wall, where fibronectin was more abundant on the luminal side and tenascin-C on the extraluminal side of the vascular BM. To note, tumor vessels were diversely positive for tenascin-C and oncofetal fibronectin, suggesting a temporally and spatially regulated expression of these ECM proteins in the tumor vasculature and may reflect different maturation states of the vessels. Re-expression of fibronectin occurs during pathological angiogenesis in various diseases such as cancer, late-stage atherosclerosis, and blinding ocular conditions [123, 124].

3. Cell-extracellular matrix interactions and angiogenesis

3.1 Integrins

Integrins are the main receptors involved in cell-matrix contacts. They contain transmembrane subunits α and β, large extracellular domain, and intracellular domain that interacts with cytoskeleton proteins. Subunits form 24 integrins. Integrins provide transmission of chemical and mechanical signals, which results in rearrangement of the cell cytoskeleton and activation of pathways that control cell survival and motility, angiogenesis, differentiation, and apoptosis. The ability of the cell to survive without contact with a substrate is a feature of tumor cells. Integrin expression changes significantly during carcinogenesis and different tumors express different integrins. Integrin α6β4 in cooperation with epidermal growth factor receptor (EGFR) is expressed mostly in breast carcinoma [125], while integrin αVβ3 in cooperation with platelet-derived growth factor (PDGF) and EGFR are expressed in glioblastomas and melanomas [126]. The role of integrins in tumor angiogenesis has been partially discussed above in relation to laminins and will also be discussed below.

Matrix metalloproteinases (MMPs), also known as matrixins, are members of the metzincin protease superfamily of zinc-endopeptidases. There are 187 members of MMPs which are encoded in the human genome and 28 members are secreted MMPs. They can degrade every protein in ECM and basement membranes. Several MMPs are membrane-type which contribute to the precise localization of protease activity, as this is required at the edge of migrating cells. Several MMPs—collagenase, gelatinase, matrilysin degrades collagen, gelatin, and fibronectin, respectively. Stromelysin degrades structural proteins and proteoglycans. MMP activity is regulated by tissue inhibitors of MMPs (TIMPs 1–4) which are produced by more cells than MMPs themselves [127]. MMPs are directly implicated in embryonic growth and tissue morphogenesis that require disruption of ECM barriers for microenvironment remodeling and cell migration and contribute to the formation of a complex microenvironment for tumor development and progression through activation of growth factors, suppression of tumor cell apoptosis, destruction of chemokine gradients developed by host immune response, or release ECM-sequestered angiogenic factors [128]. For example, MMP-11 (human stromelysin-3, hST-3) favored the release of insulin-like growth factor 1 that is bound to specific binding proteins (IGFBPs) [129].

MMP-9 can proteolytically activate TGF-β and promote tumor invasion and angiogenesis [130]. Several other pro-angiogenic factors such as VEGF and basic fibroblast growth factor (bFGF) are induced/activated by MMPs. MMP-14 overexpression by cancer cells increases VEGF synthesis and promotes angiogenesis in glioblastomas [131] and breast carcinomas [132, 133]. VEGF expression was also inspired by MMP-2 in A549 lung adenocarcinoma cells through the binding to αvβ3 and activated integrin signaling [134]. Cancer cell-derived MMP-13 (collagenase-3) also induced VEGF synthesis by endothelial cells and fibroblasts and initiated tumor angiogenesis in vivo [135]. MMP-1, -8, and -13 are collagenases associated with angiogenesis and their loss leads to irreversible rupture of the matrix [136]. The fragmentation of basement membrane type IV collagen is carried out by MMP-2 and MMP-9. Type IV collagenase activity is important in the early steps of endothelial cell morphogenesis/capillary formation. Interstitial collagenase (MMP-1) is a membrane-type 1 matrix metalloproteinase (MT1-MMP) that can also break down collagen types I–III, gelatin, laminin, and other ECM components. MT1 MMP is expressed by endothelial cells and it may regulate angiogenesis by activating pro-MMP2 and by cleaving collagens on the cell surface at a highly localized site [136]. Tissue inhibitors of metalloproteinases regulate them, playing a key role in angiogenesis regulation by inhibiting neovascularization.

3.2 Matrix topology, stiffness, and solid stress

Physical and chemical features of the tumor environment determine matrix topology (architecture) and stiffness that depends on the size of biopolymer fibers and the density of the fiber network [137]. Connective tissue is characterized by different fiber arrangements. Different combinations and densities of the cells, fibers, and other ECM components as well as different fiber arrangements ranging from loose or random to highly aligned structures, produce graded variations of connective tissue. ECM topology can represent an important regulator of cell motility through physical signals that geometrically impel adhesion foci to conduct directional migration [138]. Cancer cells perform contact guidance mediated by mechanosensory integrins through which they, using contractile force, actively remodel the ECM fibers surrounding a tumor (align them perpendicularly to the tumor) [137–139]. Dense fibrillar collagen that is characteristic of breast cancer stroma forms radial patterns extending away from tumors. On the other hand, the reticular arrangement of the collagen matrix surrounding mammary glands may anchor and/or hinder cells. Thus, ECM topography, in particular, its non-linear pattern reduces invasion while linear structure promotes it. Matrix concentration and post-translational modifications such as glycosylation and cross-linking affect the mechanical properties, including viscoelasticity or stiffness. Tumors exhibit a higher degree of stiffness than their normal adjacent counterpart. For example, the healthy mammary gland is highly compliant (elastic modulus E = ~200 Pa), while the average tumor is stiffer (E = ~4000 Pa). Both the tumor-surrounding stroma and vasculature exhibit increased stiffness (E = ~800–1000 Pa and ~450 Pa [140].

Changes in ECM topology and stiffness can shape mechanosensing events and activate intracellular signaling processes involved in cell migration. Among signaling pathways/genes involved in directionally persistent migration are, for example, vinculin, talin, FAK, p130CAS, and filamin A. Integrin receptors and the physical arrangement of adhesions assure orientation of the cytoskeleton while leading-edge protrusions can be stabilized by matrix orientation [137, 138]. When cancer cells experience an increase in ECM stiffness, they respond to the change by generating increased traction forces on their surroundings by regulating growth factor signaling and focal adhesion formation. For this purpose, the cell has several alternatives: for example, it can either force the network fibers apart and remodel the shape, form trails of variable caliber until it can pass through the pore, or the tumor cell degrades the fiber matrix via multistep pericellular proteolysis that was observed in individual and collective cancer cell migration [140]. Increased tumor tissue stiffness has been linked to tumor progression, direct stem cell differentiation, cell-cell and cell–matrix adhesion, hyaluronan synthesis, and expression of genes that play important roles in invasion and metastasis [128, 141–143]. A computational model was used to investigate the effect of ECM topography on vascular morphogenesis and explanation of mechanisms that control cell shape and orientation, sprout extension speeds, and sprout morphology. Sprout extension speed and morphology depend on matrix density, fiber network connectedness, and fiber orientation and varying matrix fiber density affect the likelihood of capillary sprout branching. The authors calculated optimal density for capillary network formation and suggested matrix heterogeneity as a mechanism for sprout branching. The density of the matrix fibers has a strong effect on the extension speed and the morphology of a new blood vessel pointing to new targets for pro- and anti-angiogenesis therapies [144].

Another important tumor characteristic is tumor growth-induced solid stress. As tumor cells proliferate they sequentially create new solid material (i.e. cells and matrix components) which pushes against the surrounding tumor microenvironment. Uncontrolled proliferation of cancer cells leads to ignorance of contact inhibition, their expansion imposes elastic tension on the surrounding tumor microenvironment, storing stress through the deformation of adaptable structures, and collapsing delicate structures, such as blood and lymphatic vessels. Interestingly, solid stress is accumulated within the tumor and is still sustained after the tumor excision [145]. Collagen and hyaluronan molecules are the main contributors of the ECM to solid stress. Collagen, as it becomes stiffer when stretched, is responsible for tensile stress. This observation is valid for both capsular and interstitial collagen. When hyaluronan resists compression, its negatively charged chains are pushed away, owing to electrostatic repulsion and trap water, therefore matrix becomes poorly compressible [145]. The compression of vessels by solid stress may create potential obstacles to drug delivery: the collapse of blood vessels hampers access to systemically administered drugs. This collapse might explain the fact that neoplasias with more ECM might be more resistant to treatment. For instance, chondrosarcomas, chordomas, or pancreatic ductal adenocarcinoma (the latter has the highest solid stress magnitude 7 kPa = 52.5 mmHg) are tumors rich in ECM and refractory to chemotherapy [146–148]. Further, the lack of lymphatic vessel function induces drainage compromise, leading to uniformly elevated interstitial fluid pressure. As a result, the transport of therapeutics, like antibodies and nanoparticles, is reduced because the dominant mode of transport becomes diffusion which is an inadequately slow process for large particles [149]. In this sense, decreasing solid stress by the angiotensin inhibitor, losartan, decompress tumor blood vessels, enhances drug delivery, and potentiates chemotherapy effects [150].

As stated above, endothelial activation is believed to be predominantly related to biochemical signals. However, mechanical forces have more recently also been demonstrated to regulate endothelial cell phenotype and function. Recent work has shown that mechanical forces control endothelial cell proliferation, survival, and migration [151, 152] and fluid shear stress from blood flow plays a critical role in regulating vessel morphogenesis, sprouting, and barrier function [153, 154]. To convert mechanical forces and biophysical signals into intracellular biochemical reaction cascades, endothelial cells employ a complex system of mechanosensors (actin cytoskeleton, integrins, cell-cell adhesion receptors, receptor tyrosine kinases, ion channels, and G-protein-coupled receptors) to sense and respond to mechanical forces [155]. Matrix stiffening enhanced integrin-mediated Rho/Rho-associated protein kinase (ROCK) activity and contraction in tumor epithelial and endothelial cells [156–158]. Tumor endothelial cells have abnormal mechanosensitivity to uniaxial cyclic strain transmitted through the ECM, which is mediated by vigorous regulation of Rho activity and cytoskeletal tension. Normal and tumor endothelial cells express similar levels of active β1 and β3 integrins [159]. Tumor endothelial cells demonstrate constitutively high baseline activity of Rho and ROCK, thicker stress fibers, higher adhesion strength, and augmented cytoskeletal tension. Logically, described features are mainly due to higher intrinsic Rho and ROCK-related cytoskeletal tension in the background of unchanged levels of integrins. These dynamics between normal and tumor endothelial cells in response to mechanical impulses suggest that the aberrant mechanical forces from the tumor microenvironment may cause tumor endothelial cells to gradually obtain an altered phenotype. Such alteration may further enable tumor endothelial cells to spread over a wider range of matrix stiffness [155, 158]. Specific integrins have been demonstrated to contribute to non-tumor and tumor angiogenesis. The expression of α1β1 and α2β1 integrins is upregulated by VEGF in endothelial cells [160], and the combined antagonism of α1β1 and α2β1 reduced human squamous cell carcinoma growth and angiogenesis [161]. The α5β1 integrin is selectively expressed in angiogenic vasculature. Upregulated αvβ3 and αvβ5 integrins in endothelial cells are necessary for the growth and survival facilitation of neovessels [162]. As already mentioned, αv integrins are also involved in cytokine-dependent pathways of angiogenesis. Integrin αvβ3 is incumbent in pathways activated by FGF or TNFα while integrin αvβ5 is necessary for angiogenic pathways activated by VEGF or TGFα [163]. Specifically, the αvβ5 integrin pathway downstream of VEGF causes activation of FAK and Src kinase [164]. The αvβ3 integrin has also been associated with VEGFR2 and the binding of αvβ3 to its corresponding ECM ligands has been shown to increase VEGF signaling [165]. Integrin αvβ3 is overexpressed in newly developed vasculature of mammary carcinoma [166], the expression level of αvβ3 and αvβ5 integrins in tumor neovessels were found to be associated with the neuroblastoma grade [167]. The experimental inhibition of αvβ3 integrin suppressed angiogenesis and related breast tumor growth in immunodeficient (SCID) mouse/human chimera [166] and resulted in tumor reduction in human clinical trials [168]. Combined inhibition of αvβ3 and αvβ5 integrins also significantly reduced growth of human melanoma xenografts in SCID mice [169]. Integrin α6β4 signaling has similarly been involved in incipient invasive phase of pathological angiogenesis. The β4 substrate domain promotes bFGF-mediated angiogenesis in matrigel plug assay and hypoxia-inducible factor VEGF-mediated angiogenesis in the retinal neovascularization model regulates sprouting angiogenesis by forced nuclear translocation of activated ERK and NF-κB in migrating endotheliocytes [170]. Furthermore, targeted deletion of the signaling domain of the integrin β4 significantly reduced the size and microvascular density in various tumors including melanoma, lung cancer, lymphoma, or fibrosarcoma [170]. These data demonstrate the role of cytoskeletal- and integrin-mediated mechanosensory pathways in facilitating tumor angiogenesis.

3.3 Hypoxia and interstitial fluid pressure

Hypoxia is another feature of the abnormal tumor microenvironment that is intrinsically linked to the formation of neovasculature and clinically manifests with metastatic progression and worse patient survival [171, 172]. Diffusion-limited hypoxia is a sequel of tumor cells located distantly from the blood-supplied areas. Such cells "suffer" from prolonged hypoxia and tumor cells are kept viable for hours to a few days in such environment [173]. Within the cell, hypoxia induces oncogenes, enhances DNA mutation chance, and selects for cells with increased apoptotic rate [171, 174]. Extracellularly, hypoxia supports tumor progression by increased matrix deposition, turnover, cross-linking, and remodeling [175]. HIF-1α increases vascularization in hypoxic areas and allows for the survival and proliferation of cancer cells, its inhibition prevents the expansion of neoplasia [176]. Along with known angiogenic factors, novel ones and their receptors include VEGF, VEGFR-1, -2, bFGF, platelet-derived growth factor B (PDGF), insulin-like growth factor II (IGF2), adrenomedullin, and epidermal growth factor (EGF) are targets of the HIF transcription factors. Several of these angiogenesis-related gene products, including iNOS, endothelin, adrenomedullin, and heme oxygenase 1, are also implicated in the modulation of local blood flow by regulating the vascular tone [177]. The well-known EMT activators such as Snail, Slug, and Twist are also induced by hypoxia [178]. Hypoxia also affects stem cells [179] that become pluripotent and aggressive with high metastatic potential. Resistance to anti-angiogenic therapy thus may be mediated by HIF-1α activated genes. Therapeutical targeting of hypoxia includes bioreductive prodrugs, HIF-1 targeting, and genetic engineering of anaerobic bacteria [180].

Abnormal metabolism in the tumor is further characterized by a decrease in extracellular pH. The known sources of H^+ ions in tumors are by- or end-products of anaerobic glycolysis, such as lactic acid and carbonic acid [181, 182]. The dysbalance between production and removal of H^+ ions lowers the extracellular pH in tumors. The level of pH also decreases in tumors with increasing distance from nearest blood vessels. Low extracellular pH causes stress-induced alteration of VEGF and IL-8 gene upregulation and relevant protein expression in three different tumor cells in vitro [183]. When the possible relationship between pH, pO2, and their effect on VEGF expression in vivo was examined using GFP imaging of tissues, pO2 and pH appear to regulate VEGF transcription in tumors independently. For example, in the hypoxic state or neutral pH, VEGF-promoter activity increased, with a decrease in pO2 and independent of pH. In decreased pH or oxygenated conditions, VEGF-promoter activity increased, with a decrease in pH and independent of pO2 [184]. To conclude, these key microenvironmental factors regulate angiogenic profiles in a complementary mode.

Another pathophysiologic feature of the tumor microenvironment is elevated interstitial fluid pressure (IFP) in the range of 10–100 mmHg [185, 186]. IFP of normal tissue is around zero [187]. The driving force in increasing tumor IFP is the tumor vasculature [188, 189]. In contrast to normal vessels which are characterized by dichotomous branching, tumor vasculature is chaotic, with trifurcations and branches with unsteady calibers, larger inter-endothelial junctions, multiple fenestrations, vesicles, vesico-vacuolar channels and a disruption of normal basement membrane [190]. Due to described ultrastructural alterations, vascular permeability in solid tumors is generally higher compared to normal counterparts. Tumors, also either lack lymphatics or the intratumoral vessels are non-functional [191], as a result, excess fluid accumulates in the interstitium resulted in elevated IFP. In IFP regulation model, fibroblasts actively regulate the tension applied to the ECM through integrins which enable fibroblasts to modify collagen fiber tension and modulate the elasticity of the ECM in response to hyaluronan and proteoglycan expansion. According to [192], interestingly, a significantly dense and stiffer collagen framework and related higher IFP is also a result of the synthesis of another important proteoglycan fibromodulin by stromal fibroblasts, which is mainly promoted by emerged inflammatory processes in malignant tumors. Interstitial fluid pressure may serve as another target for cancer therapy. Roh and colleagues [193] reported an inverse relationship between tumor IFP and degree of tissue oxygenation and suggested IFP's role in predicting radiotherapy effect. Increased tumor IFP can also act as an obstacle to drug delivery, which makes questionable their efficacy. Several studies have also demonstrated advanced amelioration of chemotherapeutics following a reduction in tumor IFP [150].

4. Conclusions

The extracellular matrix in non-tumor states regulates tissue development and homeostasis, and its deregulation imparts to neoplasia and its progression. It serves not only as the mechanical milieu upon which cells/tissues inhabit but creates and exerts critical biochemical and biomechanical messages that drive cell growth, survival, differentiation, migration, and manage neoangiogenesis and immune scaffold. The cellular mechanisms inducing both angiogenesis and immunosuppressive responses are often reached by the same cell types and soluble factors. Studies point out that combinatorial strategies toward many potential targets with emphasis on angiogenesis should be adapted as a useful therapeutic approach to hinder/reverse tumor progression.

Author details

Gvantsa Kharaishvili
Faculty of Medicine and Dentistry, Department of Clinical and Molecular Pathology, Palacky University, Olomouc, Czech Republic

*Address all correspondence to: gvantsa.kharaishvili@upol.cz

References

[1] Ayoubi S, Dunn IF, Al-Mefty O. 31—Meningiomas. In: Kaye AH, Laws ER, editors. Brain Tumors. 3rd ed. London: W.B.Saunders; 2012. pp. 600-629. ISBN 9780443069673

[2] Conti CJ. 14.16 Mechanisms of tumor progression. In: McQueen CA, editor. Comprehensive Toxicology. 2nd ed. Oxford, England: Elsevier; 2010. pp. 335-347. ISBN 9780080468846,2

[3] Liotta LA, Kohn EC. The microenvironment of the tumour-host interface. Nature. 2001;**411**(6835):375-379

[4] Anderson NM, Simon MC. The tumor microenvironment. Current Biology. 2020;**30**(16):R921-Rr25

[5] Erler JT, Weaver VM. Three-dimensional context regulation of metastasis. Clinical & Experimental Metastasis. 2009;**26**(1):35-49

[6] Järveläinen H, Sainio A, Koulu M, et al. Extracellular matrix molecules: Potential targets in pharmacotherapy. Pharmacological Reviews. 2009;**61**(2): 198-223

[7] Schulz S. C-type natriuretic peptide and guanylyl cyclase B receptor. Peptides. 2005;**26**(6):1024-1034

[8] Mescher AL, Mescher AL, Junqueira LCU. Junqueira's Basic Histology: Text and Atlas. 14th ed. New York: McGraw-Hill Education; 2016

[9] Ricard-Blum S. The collagen family. Cold Spring Harbor Perspectives in Biology. 2011;**3**(1):a004978

[10] Heino J. The collagen family members as cell adhesion proteins. BioEssays. 2007;**29**(10):1001-1010

[11] Ricard-Blum S, Ruggiero F. The collagen superfamily: From the extracellular matrix to the cell membrane. Pathologie Biologie. 2005;**53**(7):430-442

[12] Mander, Lewis N, Liu, Hung-wen. Comprehensive Natural Products II: Chemistry and Biology. Lewis Mander, Hung-Wen (Ben) Liu. The Netherlands: Elsevier Amsterdam; 2010

[13] Fleischmajer R, Perlish JS, Burgeson RE, et al. Type I and type III collagen interactions during fibrillogenesis. Annals of the New York Academy of Sciences. 1990;**580**:161-175

[14] Niyibizi C, Eyre DR. Bone type V collagen: Chain composition and location of a trypsin cleavage site. Connective Tissue Research. 1989;**20**(1-4):247-250

[15] Mayne R. Cartilage collagens. What is their function, and are they involved in articular disease? Arthritis and Rheumatism. 1989;**32**(3):241-246

[16] Bourgot I, Primac I, Louis T, et al. Reciprocal interplay between fibrillar collagens and collagen-binding integrins: Implications in cancer progression and metastasis. Frontiers in Oncology. 2020;**10**:1488

[17] Twardowski T, Fertala A, Orgel JP, et al. Type I collagen and collagen mimetics as angiogenesis promoting superpolymers. Current Pharmaceutical Design. 2007;**13**(35):3608-3621

[18] Mukwaya A, Jensen L, Lagali N. Relapse of pathological angiogenesis: Functional role of the basement membrane and potential treatment strategies. Experimental & Molecular Medicine. 2021;**53**(2):189-201

[19] Mancuso MR, Davis R, Norberg SM, et al. Rapid vascular regrowth in tumors

after reversal of VEGF inhibition. The Journal of Clinical Investigation. 2006;**116**(10):2610-2621

[20] Wu Y, Ge G. Complexity of type IV collagens: From network assembly to function. Biological Chemistry. 2019;**400**(5):565-574

[21] Khoshnoodi J, Pedchenko V, Hudson BG. Mammalian collagen IV. Microscopy Research and Technique. 2008;**71**(5):357-370

[22] Kisling A, Lust RM, Katwa LC. What is the role of peptide fragments of collagen I and IV in health and disease? Life Sciences. 2019;**228**:30-34

[23] Ricard-Blum S, Vallet SD. Fragments generated upon extracellular matrix remodeling: Biological regulators and potential drugs. Matrix Biology. 2019;**75-76**:170-189

[24] Aikio M, Alahuhta I, Nurmenniemi S, et al. Arresten, a collagen-derived angiogenesis inhibitor, suppresses invasion of squamous cell carcinoma. PLoS One. 2012;7(12):e51044

[25] Colorado PC, Torre A, Kamphaus G, et al. Anti-angiogenic cues from vascular basement membrane collagen. Cancer Research. 2000;**60**(9):2520-2526

[26] Williamson SC, Metcalf RL, Trapani F, et al. Vasculogenic mimicry in small cell lung cancer. Nature Communications. 2016;**7**:13322

[27] Chiablaem K, Lirdprapamongkol K, Keeratichamroen S, et al. Curcumin suppresses vasculogenic mimicry capacity of hepatocellular carcinoma cells through STAT3 and PI3K/AKT inhibition. Anticancer Research. 2014;**34**(4):1857-1864

[28] Chen YS, Chen ZP. Vasculogenic mimicry: A novel target for glioma therapy. Chinese Journal of Cancer. 2014;**33**(2):74-79

[29] Ma Y, Wu T, Zhou H, et al. Canstatin represses glioma growth by inhibiting formation of VM-like structures. Translational Neuroscience. 2021;**12**(1):309-319

[30] Vautrin-Glabik A, Devy J, Bour C, et al. Angiogenesis inhibition by a short 13 amino acid peptide sequence of tetrastatin, the α4(IV) NC1 domain of collagen IV. Frontiers in Cell and Development Biology. 2020;**8**:775

[31] Karagiannis ED, Popel AS. A systematic methodology for proteome-wide identification of peptides inhibiting the proliferation and migration of endothelial cells. Proceedings of the National Academy of Sciences of the United States of America. 2008;**105**(37):13775-13780

[32] Karagiannis ED, Popel AS. Identification of novel short peptides derived from the alpha 4, alpha 5, and alpha 6 fibrils of type IV collagen with anti-angiogenic properties. Biochemical and Biophysical Research Communications. 2007;**354**(2):434-439

[33] Rhodes JM, Simons M. The extracellular matrix and blood vessel formation: Not just a scaffold. Journal of Cellular and Molecular Medicine. 2007;**11**(2):176-205

[34] Baud S, Duca L, Bochicchio B, et al. Elastin peptides in aging and pathological conditions. Biomolecular Concepts. 2013;**4**(1):65-76

[35] Duca L, Floquet N, Alix AJ, et al. Elastin as a matrikine. Critical Reviews in Oncology/Hematology. 2004;**49**(3):235-244

[36] Salesse S, Odoul L, Chazée L, et al. Elastin molecular aging promotes

MDA-MB-231 breast cancer cell invasiveness. FEBS Open Bio. 2018;**8**(9):1395-1404

[37] Robinet A, Fahem A, Cauchard JH, et al. Elastin-derived peptides enhance angiogenesis by promoting endothelial cell migration and tubulogenesis through upregulation of MT1-MMP. Journal of Cell Science. 2005;**118**(Pt 2):343-356

[38] Taylor KR, Gallo RL. Glycosaminoglycans and their proteoglycans: Host-associated molecular patterns for initiation and modulation of inflammation. The FASEB Journal. 2006;**20**(1):9-22

[39] Khoshnoodi J, Cartailler JP, Alvares K, et al. Molecular recognition in the assembly of collagens: Terminal noncollagenous domains are key recognition modules in the formation of triple helical protomers. The Journal of Biological Chemistry. 2006;**281**(50):38117-38121

[40] Chen CG, Gubbiotti MA, Kapoor A, et al. Autophagic degradation of HAS2 in endothelial cells: A novel mechanism to regulate angiogenesis. Matrix Biology. 2020;**90**:1-19

[41] Heldin P, Lin CY, Kolliopoulos C, et al. Regulation of hyaluronan biosynthesis and clinical impact of excessive hyaluronan production. Matrix Biology. 2019;**78-79**:100-117

[42] Tolg C, Yuan H, Flynn SM, et al. Hyaluronan modulates growth factor induced mammary gland branching in a size dependent manner. Matrix Biology. 2017;**63**:117-132

[43] Soldevila-Barreda JJ, Romero-Canelón I, Habtemariam A, et al. Transfer hydrogenation catalysis in cells as a new approach to anticancer drug design. Nature Communications. 2015;**6**: 6582

[44] Tammi MI, Oikari S, Pasonen-Seppänen S, et al. Activated hyaluronan metabolism in the tumor matrix—Causes and consequences. Matrix Biology. 2019;**78-79**:147-164

[45] Bourguignon LYW, Earle C, Shiina M. Hyaluronan-CD44 interaction promotes HPV 16 E6 oncogene-mediated oropharyngeal cell carcinoma survival and chemoresistance. Matrix Biology. 2019;**78-79**:180-200

[46] Karalis TT, Heldin P, Vynios DH, et al. Tumor-suppressive functions of 4-MU on breast cancer cells of different ER status: Regulation of hyaluronan/HAS2/CD44 and specific matrix effectors. Matrix Biology. 2019;**78-79**:118-138

[47] Chanmee T, Ontong P, Itano N. Hyaluronan: A modulator of the tumor microenvironment. Cancer Letters. 2016;**375**(1):20-30

[48] Bernert B, Porsch H, Heldin P. Hyaluronan synthase 2 (HAS2) promotes breast cancer cell invasion by suppression of tissue metalloproteinase inhibitor 1 (TIMP-1). Journal of Biological Chemistry. 2011;**286**(49):42349-42359

[49] Caon I, Bartolini B, Parnigoni A, et al. Revisiting the hallmarks of cancer: The role of hyaluronan. Seminars in Cancer Biology. 2020;**62**:9-19

[50] Kim YH, Lee SB, Shim S, et al. Hyaluronic acid synthase 2 promotes malignant phenotypes of colorectal cancer cells through transforming growth factor beta signaling. Cancer Science. 2019;**110**(7):2226-2236

[51] Goyal A, Gubbiotti MA, Chery DR, et al. Endorepellin-evoked autophagy contributes to angiostasis. Journal of Biological Chemistry. 2016;**291**(37):19245-19256

[52] Bix G, Castello R, Burrows M, et al. Endorepellin in vivo: Targeting the tumor vasculature and retarding cancer growth and metabolism. Journal of the National Cancer Institute. 2006;**98**(22):1634-1646

[53] Folkman J. Tumor suppression by p53 is mediated in part by the antiangiogenic activity of endostatin and tumstatin. Science's STKE. 2006;**2006**(354):pe35

[54] Mantovani A, Marchesi F, Malesci A, et al. Tumour-associated macrophages as treatment targets in oncology. Nature Reviews Clinical Oncology. 2017;**14**(7):399-416

[55] Spinelli FM, Vitale DL, Icardi A, et al. Hyaluronan preconditioning of monocytes/macrophages affects their angiogenic behavior and regulation of TSG-6 expression in a tumor type-specific manner. The FEBS Journal. 2019;**286**(17):3433-3449

[56] Sokolowska M, Chen LY, Eberlein M, et al. Low molecular weight hyaluronan activates cytosolic phospholipase A2α and eicosanoid production in monocytes and macrophages. The Journal of Biological Chemistry. 2014;**289**(7):4470-4488

[57] Rayahin JE, Buhrman JS, Zhang Y, et al. High and low molecular weight hyaluronic acid differentially influence macrophage activation. ACS Biomaterials Science & Engineering. 2015;**1**(7):481-493

[58] Cattaruzza S, Perris R. Proteoglycan control of cell movement during wound healing and cancer spreading. Matrix Biology. 2005;**24**(6):400-417

[59] Murdoch AD, Iozzo RV. Prokaryotic expression of proteoglycans. Methods in Molecular Biology. 2001;**171**:231-238

[60] Iozzo RV, Murdoch AD. Proteoglycans of the extracellular environment: Clues from the gene and protein side offer novel perspectives in molecular diversity and function. The FASEB Journal. 1996;**10**(5):598-614

[61] Iozzo RV. The family of the small leucine-rich proteoglycans: Key regulators of matrix assembly and cellular growth. Critical Reviews in Biochemistry and Molecular Biology. 1997;**32**(2):141-174

[62] Chen S, Young MF, Chakravarti S, et al. Interclass small leucine-rich repeat proteoglycan interactions regulate collagen fibrillogenesis and corneal stromal assembly. Matrix Biology. 2014;**35**:103-111

[63] Reese SP, Underwood CJ, Weiss JA. Effects of decorin proteoglycan on fibrillogenesis, ultrastructure, and mechanics of type I collagen gels. Matrix Biology. 2013;**32**(7-8):414-423

[64] Schaefer L, Iozzo RV. Small leucine-rich proteoglycans, at the crossroad of cancer growth and inflammation. Current Opinion in Genetics & Development. 2012;**22**(1):56-57

[65] Järveläinen H, Sainio A, Wight TN. Pivotal role for decorin in angiogenesis. Matrix Biology. 2015;**43**:15-26

[66] Goyal A, Neill T, Owens RT, et al. Decorin activates AMPK, an energy sensor kinase, to induce autophagy in endothelial cells. Matrix Biology. 2014;**34**:46-54

[67] Neill T, Schaefer L, Iozzo RV. Decorin: A guardian from the matrix. The American Journal of Pathology. 2012;**181**(2):380-387

[68] Santra M, Reed CC, Iozzo RV. Decorin binds to a narrow region of the epidermal growth factor (EGF) receptor, partially overlapping but

distinct from the EGF-binding epitope. The Journal of Biological Chemistry. 2002;**277**(38):35671-35681

[69] Schlessinger J. Ligand-induced, receptor-mediated dimerization and activation of EGF receptor. Cell. 2002;**110**(6):669-672

[70] Zhu JX, Goldoni S, Bix G, et al. Decorin evokes protracted internalization and degradation of the epidermal growth factor receptor via caveolar endocytosis. The Journal of Biological Chemistry. 2005;**280**(37):32468-32479

[71] Moreth K, Iozzo RV, Schaefer L. Small leucine-rich proteoglycans orchestrate receptor crosstalk during inflammation. Cell Cycle. 2012;**11**(11):2084-2091

[72] Buraschi S, Pal N, Tyler-Rubinstein N, et al. Decorin antagonizes Met receptor activity and down-regulates {beta}-catenin and Myc levels. The Journal of Biological Chemistry. 2010;**285**(53):42075-42085

[73] Danilkovitch-Miagkova A, Miagkov A, Skeel A, et al. Oncogenic mutants of RON and MET receptor tyrosine kinases cause activation of the beta-catenin pathway. Molecular and Cellular Biology. 2001;**21**(17):5857-5868

[74] Kharaishvili G, Simkova D, Makharoblidze E, et al. Wnt signaling in prostate development and carcinogenesis. Biomedical Papers of the Medical Faculty of the University Palacky, Olomouc, Czech Republic. 2011;**155**(1):11-18

[75] Rasola A, Fassetta M, De Bacco F, et al. A positive feedback loop between hepatocyte growth factor receptor and beta-catenin sustains colorectal cancer cell invasive growth. Oncogene. 2007;**26**(7):1078-1087

[76] Kasprzak A. Angiogenesis-related functions of Wnt signaling in colorectal carcinogenesis. Cancers. 2020;**12**(12):3601

[77] Asano K, Nelson CM, Nandadasa S, et al. Stromal versican regulates tumor growth by promoting angiogenesis. Scientific Reports. 2017;**7**(1):17225

[78] Ricciardelli C, Russell DL, Ween MP, et al. Formation of hyaluronan- and versican-rich pericellular matrix by prostate cancer cells promotes cell motility. The Journal of Biological Chemistry. 2007;**282**(14):10814-10825

[79] Wight TN. Versican: A versatile extracellular matrix proteoglycan in cell biology. Current Opinion in Cell Biology. 2002;**14**(5):617-623

[80] Wight TN, Kinsella MG, Evanko SP, et al. Versican and the regulation of cell phenotype in disease. Biochimica et Biophysica Acta. 2014;**1840**(8):2441-2451

[81] Nandadasa S, Foulcer S, Apte SS. The multiple, complex roles of versican and its proteolytic turnover by ADAMTS proteases during embryogenesis. Matrix Biology. 2014;**35**:34-41

[82] Yang W, Yee AJ. Versican V2 isoform enhances angiogenesis by regulating endothelial cell activities and fibronectin expression. FEBS Letters. 2013;**587**(2):185-192

[83] Lin H, Wilson JE, Roberts CR, et al. Biglycan, decorin, and versican protein expression patterns in coronary arteriopathy of human cardiac allograft: Distinctness as compared to native atherosclerosis. The Journal of Heart and Lung Transplantation. 1996;**15**(12):1233-1247

[84] Dutt S, Kléber M, Matasci M, et al. Versican V0 and V1 guide migratory

neural crest cells. The Journal of Biological Chemistry. 2006;**281**(17): 12123-12131

[85] Yamagata M, Kimata K. Repression of a malignant cell-substratum adhesion phenotype by inhibiting the production of the anti-adhesive proteoglycan, PG-M/versican. Journal of Cell Science. 1994;**107**(Pt 9):2581-2590

[86] Paulus W, Baur I, Dours-Zimmermann MT, et al. Differential expression of versican isoforms in brain tumors. Journal of Neuropathology and Experimental Neurology. 1996;**55**(5):528-533

[87] Koyama H, Hibi T, Isogai Z, et al. Hyperproduction of hyaluronan in neu-induced mammary tumor accelerates angiogenesis through stromal cell recruitment: Possible involvement of versican/PG-M. The American Journal of Pathology. 2007;**170**(3):1086-1099

[88] Masui T, Hosotani R, Tsuji S, et al. Expression of METH-1 and METH-2 in pancreatic cancer. Clinical Cancer Research. 2001;**7**(11):3437-3443

[89] Fernández-Rodríguez R, Rodríguez-Baena FJ, Martino-Echarri E, et al. Stroma-derived but not tumor ADAMTS1 is a main driver of tumor growth and metastasis. Oncotarget. 2016;**7**(23):34507-34519

[90] Vázquez F, Hastings G, Ortega MA, et al. METH-1, a human ortholog of ADAMTS-1, and METH-2 are members of a new family of proteins with angio-inhibitory activity. The Journal of Biological Chemistry. 1999;**274**(33):23349-23357

[91] Reynolds LE, Watson AR, Baker M, et al. Tumour angiogenesis is reduced in the Tc1 mouse model of Down's syndrome. Nature. 2010;**465**(7299):813-817

[92] Casal C, Torres-Collado AX, Plaza-Calonge Mdel C, et al. ADAMTS1 contributes to the acquisition of an endothelial-like phenotype in plastic tumor cells. Cancer Research. 2010;**70**(11):4676-4686

[93] Ricciardelli C, Frewin KM, Tan Ide A, et al. The ADAMTS1 protease gene is required for mammary tumor growth and metastasis. The American Journal of Pathology. 2011;**179**(6):3075-3085

[94] Lu X, Wang Q, Hu G, et al. ADAMTS1 and MMP1 proteolytically engage EGF-like ligands in an osteolytic signaling cascade for bone metastasis. Genes & Development. 2009;**23**(16):1882-1894

[95] Lima MA, Dos Santos L, Turri JA, et al. Prognostic value of ADAMTS proteases and their substrates in epithelial ovarian cancer. Pathobiology. 2016;**83**(6):316-326

[96] Henry SP, Takanosu M, Boyd TC, et al. Expression pattern and gene characterization of asporin. A newly discovered member of the leucine-rich repeat protein family. The Journal of Biological Chemistry. 2001;**276**(15):12212-12221

[97] Lorenzo P, Aspberg A, Onnerfjord P, et al. Identification and characterization of asporin. A novel member of the leucine-rich repeat protein family closely related to decorin and biglycan. The Journal of Biological Chemistry. 2001;**276**(15):12201-12211

[98] Nakajima M, Kizawa H, Saitoh M, et al. Mechanisms for asporin function and regulation in articular cartilage. The Journal of Biological Chemistry. 2007;**282**(44):32185-32192

[99] Kalamajski S, Aspberg A, Lindblom K, et al. Asporin competes

with decorin for collagen binding, binds calcium and promotes osteoblast collagen mineralization. The Biochemical Journal. 2009;**423**(1):53-59

[100] Turashvili G, Bouchal J, Baumforth K, et al. Novel markers for differentiation of lobular and ductal invasive breast carcinomas by laser microdissection and microarray analysis. BMC Cancer. 2007;7:55

[101] Simkova D, Kharaishvili G, Slabakova E, et al. Glycoprotein asporin as a novel player in tumour microenvironment and cancer progression. Biomedical Papers of the Medical Faculty of the University Palacky, Olomouc, Czech Republic. 2016;**160**(4):467-473

[102] Simkova D, Kharaishvili G, Korinkova G, et al. The dual role of asporin in breast cancer progression. Oncotarget. 2016;7(32):52045-52060

[103] Turtoi A, Musmeci D, Wang Y, et al. Identification of novel accessible proteins bearing diagnostic and therapeutic potential in human pancreatic ductal adenocarcinoma. Journal of Proteome Research. 2011;**10**(9):4302-4313

[104] Orr B, Riddick AC, Stewart GD, et al. Identification of stromally expressed molecules in the prostate by tag-profiling of cancer-associated fibroblasts, normal fibroblasts and fetal prostate. Oncogene. 2012;**31**(9):1130-1142

[105] Zhan S, Li J, Ge W. Multifaceted roles of asporin in cancer: Current understanding. Frontiers in Oncology. 2019;**9**:948

[106] Sasaki T, Fässler R, Hohenester E. Laminin: The crux of basement membrane assembly. The Journal of Cell Biology. 2004;**164**(7): 959-963

[107] Patarroyo M, Tryggvason K, Virtanen I. Laminin isoforms in tumor invasion, angiogenesis and metastasis. Seminars in Cancer Biology. 2002;**12**(3):197-207

[108] Dixelius J, Jakobsson L, Genersch E, et al. Laminin-1 promotes angiogenesis in synergy with fibroblast growth factor by distinct regulation of the gene and protein expression profile in endothelial cells. The Journal of Biological Chemistry. 2004;**279**(22):23766-23772

[109] Doi M, Thyboll J, Kortesmaa J, et al. Production, purification, and migration-promoting activity on vascular endothelial cells. The Journal of Biological Chemistry. 2002;**277**(15):12741-12748

[110] Jeon H, Ono M, Kumagai C, et al. Pericytes from microvessel fragment produce type IV collagen and multiple laminin isoforms. Bioscience, Biotechnology, and Biochemistry. 1996;**60**(5):856-861

[111] Lugassy C, Shahsafaei A, Bonitz P, et al. Tumor microvessels in melanoma express the beta-2 chain of laminin. Implications for melanoma metastasis. Journal of Cutaneous Pathology. 1999;**26**(5):222-226

[112] Lugassy C, Eyden BP, Christensen L, et al. Angio-tumoral complex in human malignant melanoma characterised by free laminin: Ultrastructural and immunohistochemical observations. Journal of Submicroscopic Cytology and Pathology. 1997;**29**(1):19-28

[113] Miner JH, Patton BL, Lentz SI, et al. The laminin alpha chains: Expression, developmental transitions, and chromosomal locations of alpha1-5, identification of heterotrimeric laminins 8-11, and cloning of a novel alpha3 isoform. The Journal of Cell Biology. 1997;**137**(3):685-701

[114] Paku S, Döme B, Tóth R, et al. Organ-specificity of the extravasation process: An ultrastructural study. Clinical & Experimental Metastasis. 2000;**18**(6):481-492

[115] Kariya Y, Mori T, Yasuda C, et al. Localization of laminin alpha3B chain in vascular and epithelial basement membranes of normal human tissues and its down-regulation in skin cancers. Journal of Molecular Histology. 2008;**39**(4):435-446

[116] Mao Y, Schwarzbauer JE. Fibronectin fibrillogenesis, a cell-mediated matrix assembly process. Matrix Biology. 2005;**24**(6):389-399

[117] Vouret-Craviari V, Boulter E, Grall D, et al. ILK is required for the assembly of matrix-forming adhesions and capillary morphogenesis in endothelial cells. Journal of Cell Science. 2004;**117**(Pt 19):4559-4569

[118] Gerhardt H, Golding M, Fruttiger M, et al. VEGF guides angiogenic sprouting utilizing endothelial tip cell filopodia. The Journal of Cell Biology. 2003;**161**(6):1163-1177

[119] Uemura A, Kusuhara S, Wiegand SJ, et al. Tlx acts as a proangiogenic switch by regulating extracellular assembly of fibronectin matrices in retinal astrocytes. The Journal of Clinical Investigation. 2006;**116**(2):369-377

[120] Bazigou E, Xie S, Chen C, et al. Integrin-alpha9 is required for fibronectin matrix assembly during lymphatic valve morphogenesis. Developmental Cell. 2009;**17**(2):175-186

[121] Garmy-Susini B, Avraamides CJ, Schmid MC, et al. Integrin alpha4beta1 signaling is required for lymphangiogenesis and tumor metastasis. Cancer Research. 2010;**70**(8):3042-3051

[122] Van Obberghen-Schilling E, Tucker RP, Saupe F, et al. Fibronectin and tenascin-C: Accomplices in vascular morphogenesis during development and tumor growth. The International Journal of Developmental Biology. 2011;**55**(4-5):511-525

[123] Astrof S, Hynes RO. Fibronectins in vascular morphogenesis. Angiogenesis. 2009;**12**(2):165-175

[124] Neri D, Bicknell R. Tumour vascular targeting. Nature Reviews. Cancer. 2005;**5**(6):436-446

[125] Soung YH, Chung J. Curcumin inhibition of the functional interaction between integrin $\alpha6\beta4$ and the epidermal growth factor receptor. Molecular Cancer Therapeutics. 2011;**10**(5):883-891

[126] Desgrosellier JS, Cheresh DA. Integrins in cancer: Biological implications and therapeutic opportunities. Nature Reviews. Cancer. 2010;**10**(1):9-22

[127] Zucker S, Hymowitz M, Conner CE, et al. Rapid trafficking of membrane type 1-matrix metalloproteinase to the cell surface regulates progelatinase a activation. Laboratory Investigation. 2002;**82**(12):1673-1684

[128] Folgueras AR, Pendás AM, Sánchez LM, et al. Matrix metalloproteinases in cancer: From new functions to improved inhibition strategies. The International Journal of Developmental Biology. 2004;**48**(5-6):411-424

[129] Mañes S, Mira E, Barbacid MM, et al. Identification of insulin-like growth factor-binding protein-1 as a potential physiological substrate for human stromelysin-3. The Journal of Biological Chemistry. 1997;**272**(41):25706-25712

[130] Yu Q, Stamenkovic I. Cell surface-localized matrix metalloproteinase-9

proteolytically activates TGF-beta and promotes tumor invasion and angiogenesis. Genes & Development. 2000;**14**(2):163-176

[131] Deryugina EI, Quigley JP. Tumor angiogenesis: MMP-mediated induction of intravasation-and metastasis-sustaining neovasculature. Matrix Biology. 2015;**44-46**:94-112

[132] Sounni NE, Devy L, Hajitou A, et al. MT1-MMP expression promotes tumor growth and angiogenesis through an up-regulation of vascular endothelial growth factor expression. The FASEB Journal. 2002;**16**(6):555-564

[133] Sounni NE, Roghi C, Chabottaux V, et al. Up-regulation of vascular endothelial growth factor-A by active membrane-type 1 matrix metalloproteinase through activation of Src-tyrosine kinases. The Journal of Biological Chemistry. 2004;**279**(14):13564-13574

[134] Chetty C, Lakka SS, Bhoopathi P, et al. MMP-2 alters VEGF expression via alphaVbeta3 integrin-mediated PI3K/AKT signaling in A549 lung cancer cells. International Journal of Cancer. 2010;**127**(5):1081-1095

[135] Kudo Y, Iizuka S, Yoshida M, et al. Matrix metalloproteinase-13 (MMP-13) directly and indirectly promotes tumor angiogenesis. The Journal of Biological Chemistry. 2012;**287**(46):38716-38728

[136] Sang QX. Complex role of matrix metalloproteinases in angiogenesis. Cell Research. 1998;**8**(3):171-177

[137] Brábek J, Mierke CT, Rösel D, et al. The role of the tissue microenvironment in the regulation of cancer cell motility and invasion. Cell Communication and Signaling: CCS. 2010;**8**:22

[138] Petrie RJ, Doyle AD, Yamada KM. Random versus directionally persistent cell migration. Nature Reviews. Molecular Cell Biology. 2009;**10**(8):538-549

[139] Kraning-Rush CM, Reinhart-King CA. Controlling matrix stiffness and topography for the study of tumor cell migration. Cell Adhesion & Migration. 2012;**6**(3):274-279

[140] Kharaishvili G, Simkova D, Bouchalova, et al. The role of cancer-associated fibroblasts, solid stress and other microenvironmental factors in tumor progression and therapy resistance. Cancer Cell International. 2014;**14**:41

[141] Levental KR, Yu H, Kass L, et al. Matrix crosslinking forces tumor progression by enhancing integrin signaling. Cell. 2009;**139**(5):891-906

[142] Palumbo A Jr, Meireles Da Costa N, et al. Esophageal cancer development: Crucial clues arising from the extracellular matrix. Cell. 2020;**9**(2):455

[143] Reinhart-King CA. How matrix properties control the self-assembly and maintenance of tissues. Annals of Biomedical Engineering. 2011;**39**(7):1849-1856

[144] Bauer AL, Jackson TL, Jiang Y. Topography of extracellular matrix mediates vascular morphogenesis and migration speeds in angiogenesis. PLoS Computational Biology. 2009;**5**(7):e1000445

[145] Stylianopoulos T, Martin JD, Chauhan VP, et al. Causes, consequences, and remedies for growth-induced solid stress in murine and human tumors. Proceedings of the National Academy of Sciences of the United States of America. 2012;**109**(38):15101-15108

[146] Provenzano PP, Cuevas C, Chang AE, et al. Enzymatic targeting

of the stroma ablates physical barriers to treatment of pancreatic ductal adenocarcinoma. Cancer Cell. 2012;**21**(3):418-429

[147] Olive KP, Jacobetz MA, Davidson CJ, et al. Inhibition of Hedgehog signaling enhances delivery of chemotherapy in a mouse model of pancreatic cancer. Science. 2009;**324**(5933):1457-1461

[148] Chauhan VP, Martin JD, Liu H, et al. Angiotensin inhibition enhances drug delivery and potentiates chemotherapy by decompressing tumour blood vessels. Nature Communications. 2013;**4**:2516

[149] Honn KV, Tang DG. Adhesion molecules and tumor cell interaction with endothelium and subendothelial matrix. Cancer Metastasis Reviews. 1992;**11**(3-4):353-375

[150] Horino Y, Takahashi S, Miura T, et al. Prolonged hypoxia accelerates the posttranscriptional process of collagen synthesis in cultured fibroblasts. Life Sciences. 2002;**71**(26):3031-3045

[151] Li S, Huang NF, Hsu S. Mechanotransduction in endothelial cell migration. Journal of Cellular Biochemistry. 2005;**96**(6):1110-1126

[152] Li YS, Haga JH, Chien S. Molecular basis of the effects of shear stress on vascular endothelial cells. Journal of Biomechanics. 2005;**38**(10):1949-1971

[153] Kutys ML, Chen CS. Forces and mechanotransduction in 3D vascular biology. Current Opinion in Cell Biology. 2016;**42**:73-79

[154] Conway DE, Breckenridge MT, Hinde E, et al. Fluid shear stress on endothelial cells modulates mechanical tension across VE-cadherin and PECAM-1. Current Biology. 2013;**23**(11):1024-1030

[155] Zanotelli MR, Reinhart-King CA. Mechanical forces in tumor angiogenesis. Advances in Experimental Medicine and Biology. 2018;**1092**:91-112

[156] Paszek MJ, Zahir N, Johnson KR, et al. Tensional homeostasis and the malignant phenotype. Cancer Cell. 2005;**8**(3):241-254

[157] Paszek MJ, Weaver VM. The tension mounts: Mechanics meets morphogenesis and malignancy. Journal of Mammary Gland Biology and Neoplasia. 2004;**9**(4):325-342

[158] Ghosh K, Thodeti CK, Dudley AC, et al. Tumor-derived endothelial cells exhibit aberrant Rho-mediated mechanosensing and abnormal angiogenesis in vitro. Proceedings of the National Academy of Sciences of the United States of America. 2008;**105**(32):11305-11310

[159] Tzima E, del Pozo MA, Shattil SJ, et al. Activation of integrins in endothelial cells by fluid shear stress mediates Rho-dependent cytoskeletal alignment. The EMBO Journal. 2001;**20**(17):4639-4647

[160] Senger DR, Claffey KP, Benes JE, et al. Angiogenesis promoted by vascular endothelial growth factor: Regulation through alpha1beta1 and alpha2beta1 integrins. Proceedings of the National Academy of Sciences of the United States of America. 1997;**94**(25):13612-13617

[161] Senger DR, Perruzzi CA, Streit M, et al. The alpha(1)beta(1) and alpha(2) beta(1) integrins provide critical support for vascular endothelial growth factor signaling, endothelial cell migration, and tumor angiogenesis. The American Journal of Pathology. 2002;**160**(1):195-204

[162] Weis SM, Cheresh DA. αV integrins in angiogenesis and cancer. Cold Spring

Harbor Perspectives in Medicine. 2011;**1**(1):a006478

[163] Friedlander M, Brooks PC, Shaffer RW, et al. Definition of two angiogenic pathways by distinct alpha v integrins. Science. 1995;**270**(5241):1500-1502

[164] Hood JD, Frausto R, Kiosses WB, et al. Differential alphav integrin-mediated Ras-ERK signaling during two pathways of angiogenesis. The Journal of Cell Biology. 2003;**162**(5):933-943

[165] Soldi R, Mitola S, Strasly M, et al. Role of alphavbeta3 integrin in the activation of vascular endothelial growth factor receptor-2. The EMBO Journal. 1999;**18**(4):882-892

[166] Brooks PC, Strömblad S, Klemke R, et al. Antiintegrin alpha v beta 3 blocks human breast cancer growth and angiogenesis in human skin. The Journal of Clinical Investigation. 1995;**96**(4):1815-1822

[167] Erdreich-Epstein A, Shimada H, Groshen S, et al. Integrins alpha(v)beta3 and alpha(v)beta5 are expressed by endothelium of high-risk neuroblastoma and their inhibition is associated with increased endogenous ceramide. Cancer Research. 2000;**60**(3):712-721

[168] Eliceiri BP, Cheresh DA. The role of alphav integrins during angiogenesis: Insights into potential mechanisms of action and clinical development. The Journal of Clinical Investigation. 1999;**103**(9):1227-1230

[169] Kumar CC, Malkowski M, Yin Z, et al. Inhibition of angiogenesis and tumor growth by SCH221153, a dual alpha(v)beta3 and alpha(v)beta5 integrin receptor antagonist. Cancer Research. 2001;**61**(5):2232-2238

[170] Nikolopoulos SN, Blaikie P, Yoshioka T, et al. Integrin beta4 signaling promotes tumor angiogenesis. Cancer Cell. 2004;**6**(5):471-483

[171] Lunt SJ, Chaudary N, Hill RP. The tumor microenvironment and metastatic disease. Clinical & Experimental Metastasis. 2009;**26**(1):19-34

[172] Grum-Schwensen B, Klingelhofer J, Berg CH, et al. Suppression of tumor development and metastasis formation in mice lacking the S100A4(mts1) gene. Cancer Research. 2005;**65**(9):3772-3780

[173] Sutherland RM, Franko AJ. On the nature of the radiobiologically hypoxic fraction in tumors. International Journal of Radiation Oncology, Biology, Physics. 1980;**6**(1):117-120

[174] Duff MD, Mestre J, Maddali S, et al. Analysis of gene expression in the tumor-associated macrophage. The Journal of Surgical Research. 2007;**142**(1):119-128

[175] Helmlinger G, Sckell A, Dellian M, et al. Acid production in glycolysis-impaired tumors provides new insights into tumor metabolism. Clinical Cancer Research. 2002;**8**(4):1284-1291

[176] Schauer IG, Sood AK, Mok S, et al. Cancer-associated fibroblasts and their putative role in potentiating the initiation and development of epithelial ovarian cancer. Neoplasia. 2011;**13**(5):393-405

[177] Bagley RG. Endosialin: From vascular target to biomarker for human sarcomas. Biomarkers in Medicine. 2009;**3**(5):589-604

[178] Sun S, Ning X, Zhang Y, et al. Hypoxia-inducible factor-1alpha induces twist expression in tubular epithelial cells subjected to hypoxia, leading to epithelial-to-mesenchymal transition. Kidney International. 2009;**75**(12):1278-1287

[179] Keith B, Simon MC. Hypoxia-inducible factors, stem cells, and cancer. Cell. 2007;**129**(3):465-472

[180] Sun JD, Liu Q, Wang J, et al. Selective tumor hypoxia targeting by hypoxia-activated prodrug TH-302 inhibits tumor growth in preclinical models of cancer. Clinical Cancer Research. 2012;**18**(3):758-770

[181] Garin-Chesa P, Old LJ, Rettig WJ. Cell surface glycoprotein of reactive stromal fibroblasts as a potential antibody target in human epithelial cancers. Proceedings of the National Academy of Sciences of the United States of America. 1990;**87**(18):7235-7239

[182] Pouysségur J, Mechta-Grigoriou F. Redox regulation of the hypoxia-inducible factor. Biological Chemistry. 2006;**387**(10-11):1337-1346

[183] Xu L, Fukumura D, Jain RK. Acidic extracellular pH induces vascular endothelial growth factor (VEGF) in human glioblastoma cells via ERK1/2 MAPK signaling pathway: Mechanism of low pH-induced VEGF. The Journal of Biological Chemistry. 2002;**277**(13):11368-11374

[184] Fukumura D, Xu L, Chen Y, et al. Hypoxia and acidosis independently up-regulate vascular endothelial growth factor transcription in brain tumors in vivo. Cancer Research. 2001;**61**(16):6020-6024

[185] Nathanson SD, Nelson L. Interstitial fluid pressure in breast cancer, benign breast conditions, and breast parenchyma. Annals of Surgical Oncology. 1994;**1**(4):333-338

[186] Milosevic M, Fyles A, Hedley D, et al. Interstitial fluid pressure predicts survival in patients with cervix cancer independent of clinical prognostic factors and tumor oxygen measurements. Cancer Research. 2001;**61**(17):6400-6405

[187] Erler JT, Cawthorne CJ, Williams KJ, et al. Hypoxia-mediated down-regulation of Bid and Bax in tumors occurs via hypoxia-inducible factor 1-dependent and -independent mechanisms and contributes to drug resistance. Molecular and Cellular Biology. 2004;**24**(7):2875-2889

[188] Lunt SJ, Kalliomaki TM, Brown A, et al. Interstitial fluid pressure, vascularity and metastasis in ectopic, orthotopic and spontaneous tumours. BMC Cancer. 2008;**8**:2

[189] Jain RK, Tong RT, Munn LL. Effect of vascular normalization by antiangiogenic therapy on interstitial hypertension, peritumor edema, and lymphatic metastasis: Insights from a mathematical model. Cancer Research. 2007;**67**(6):2729-2735

[190] Winkler F, Kozin SV, Tong RT, et al. Kinetics of vascular normalization by VEGFR2 blockade governs brain tumor response to radiation: Role of oxygenation, angiopoietin-1, and matrix metalloproteinases. Cancer Cell. 2004;**6**(6):553-563

[191] Padera TP, Kadambi A, di Tomaso E, et al. Lymphatic metastasis in the absence of functional intratumor lymphatics. Science. 2002;**296**(5574):1883-1886

[192] Oldberg A, Kalamajski S, Salnikov AV, et al. Collagen-binding proteoglycan fibromodulin can determine stroma matrix structure and fluid balance in experimental carcinoma. Proceedings of the National Academy of Sciences of the United States of America. 2007;**104**(35):13966-13971

[193] Roh HD, Boucher Y, Kalnicki S, et al. Interstitial hypertension in carcinoma of uterine cervix in patients: Possible correlation with tumor oxygenation and radiation response. Cancer Research. 1991;**51**(24):6695-6698